Sex Secrets of an American Geisha

Advance praise for
Sex Secrets of an American Geisha

"You may want to wear gloves as you read *Sex Secrets of an American Geisha*—it's that HOT! The secrets of this 1st-class pleasure seekers' guide for women will reveal the intimate details you can use to unleash your own hidden desires. It'll take you and your Good Man on a trip to Paradise."

— Larry James, www.CelebrateIntimacy.com
Author of *Red Hot Love Notes for Lovers*

"Py Kim Conant provides a precious gift to readers—permission to embrace their femininity and open up to exquisite sensual possibilities. *Sex Secrets of an American Geisha* is a rare combination of self-growth, relationship, and sexual "how-to's" that educate and enlighten. Most of all it offers hope."

— Elayne Savage, Ph.D., Professional speaker, relationship coach, and author of *Breathing Room—Creating Space to Be a Couple* and *Don't Take It Personally! The Art of Dealing with Rejection* (www.QueenofRejection.com)

"A fascinating read with a truly unique perspective."

— Lisa Daily, syndicated columnist, media personality, and author of *Stop Getting Dumped!*

More advance praise for *Sex Secrets of an American Geisha*

"Conant shows us how East meets West in dating and relationships leading to marriage and really tells it like it is! This is an exciting new perspective on an age-old subject. A must read for every Motivated to Marry™ woman!

— Amy Schoen, life coach, speaker and author of *Motivated to Marry™—Now There Is a Better Method to Dating and Relationships!* (www.motivatedtomarry.com)

"The wisdom of the Asian Geisha in terms of beauty, eroticism, and pleasing high-powered men is well-known around the world. In *Sex Secrets of an American Geisha,* author Py Kim Conant imparts some of that special sexual wisdom with a Western twist and a personable style. If you want to learn to be more feminine, read this book. Great section on female ejaculation, too!"

— Susan M. Block, Ph.D., author of *The 10 Commandments of Pleasure* and producer of *Dr. Suzy's Squirt Salon: Secrets of Female Ejaculation*

"*Sex Secrets of an American Geisha* takes an intriguing and thought-provoking look at the goal of obtaining mutually loving and satisfying experiences within a committed, monogamous relationship. The author shares with us her system of actions and awareness that has so successfully contributed to her own sexual image of herself and deep appreciation of her "Good Man." Women who are hoping to find a "good" man will definitely welcome this new and refreshing approach to dating. Married women who desire a more erotic and sexual relationship with their spouse and have the desire to please their partner will find that this book is filled with advice and suggestions that can be playfully incorporated into their lives."

— Debra Burrell, CSW, psychotherapist, New York

More advance praise for *Sex Secrets of an American Geisha*

"A superb book for recapturing the essence of femininity and illuminating how its secrets can be used for not only exquisite erotic play, but for achieving a higher state of intimacy and even enlightenment."

— Deborah Sundahl, sex educator and author of *Female Ejaculation and the G-Spot*

"A fun and fascinating read! Inspiring to any woman who has ever found herself dateless on a Saturday night, this sexy how-to-find-and-keep-a-man manual will rev up your mojo and give you the confidence you need to jump into the dating pool."

— Jina Bacarr, author of *The Blonde Geisha* and *The Japanese Art of Sex*

DEDICATION

For my Good Man, Richard

ORDERING

Trade bookstores in the U.S. and Canada please contact:

Publishers Group West
1700 Fourth Street, Berkeley CA 94710
Phone: (800) 788-3123 Fax: (510) 528-3444

Hunter House books are available at bulk discounts for textbook course adoptions; to qualifying community, health-care, and government organizations; and for special promotions and fund-raising. For details please contact:

Special Sales Department
Hunter House Inc., PO Box 2914, Alameda CA 94501-0914
Phone: (510) 865-5282 Fax: (510) 865-4295
E-mail: ordering@hunterhouse.com

Individuals can order our books from most bookstores, by calling **(800) 266-5592,** or from our website at **www.hunterhouse.com**

Sex Secrets of an American Geisha

How to Attract, Satisfy and Keep Your Man

Py Kim Conant

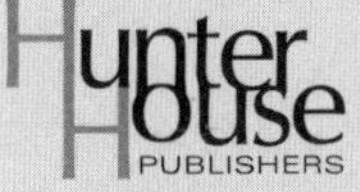

Hunter House Inc., Publishers
PO Box 2914
Alameda CA 94501-0914

LIBRARY OF CONGRESS CATALOGING-IN-PUBLICATION DATA

Conant, Py Kim.
Sex secrets of an American geisha : how to attract, satisfy and keep your man / Py Kim Conant.
p. cm. — (Positively sexual)
ISBN-13: 978-0-89793-490-9
ISBN-10: 0-89793-490-3
1. Sex instruction for women. 2. Asian American women—Sexual behavior. I. Title.
HQ46.C68 2006
613.9'6082—dc22 2006020507

PROJECT CREDITS

Cover Design: Brian Dittmar Graphic Design
Book Production: Hunter House; Blair Cavagrotti
Developmental and Copy Editor: Kelley Blewster
Proofreader: Herman Leung
Indexer: Candace Hyatt
Acquisitions Editor: Jeanne Brondino
Editor: Alexandra Mummery
Senior Marketing Associate: Reina Santana
Marketing Assistant: Liz Heck
Customer Service Manager: Christina Sverdrup
Order Fulfillment: Washul Lakdhon
Administrator: Theresa Nelson
Computer Support: Peter Eichelberger
Publisher: Kiran S. Rana

Printed and Bound by Bang Printing, Brainerd, Minnesota
Manufactured in the United States of America

9 8 7 6 5 4 3 2 1 First Edition 07 08 09 10 11

Contents

Important Note

The material in this book is intended to provide a review of information regarding relationships and sexuality. Every effort has been made to provide accurate and dependable information. The publisher, author, and editors, as well as others quoted in the book, cannot be held responsible for any error, omission, or dated material. The author and publisher assume no responsibility for any outcome of applying the information in this book in a program of self-care or under the care of a licensed practitioner. If you have questions concerning your sexual health, or about the application of the information described in this book, consult a qualified professional.

A Few Words Before We Get Started

Sex Secrets of an American Geisha is about discovering and experiencing your beauty, femininity, and sexuality while on a journey to love and marriage with a Good Man. The journey starts *today,* as you read right now. This book offers you the practical, realistic, sometimes outrageous, hot, and sexy secrets of the Far East. I pass these secrets on to you in my role of bringing Asian Geisha relationship wisdom to the women of America. I'll be your American Geisha "Older Sister" as you, my dear "Younger Sister," learn to develop a Geisha Consciousness toward what I call your "Good Man." In using these American Geisha secrets to marry your Good Man within twelve to eighteen months, you will yourself become an American Geisha.

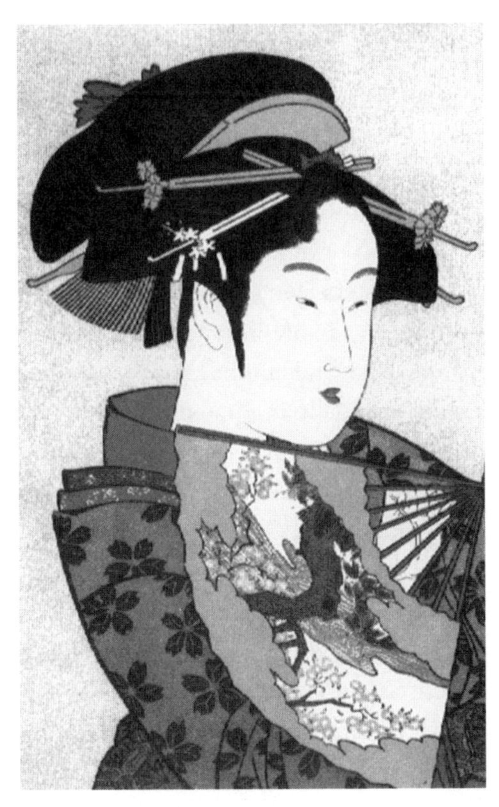

INTRODUCTION

Your Journey to Becoming an American Geisha Begins

My mind said, "I am hot and sexy. And wet." But I worried about expressing this to men because I was not expected to speak or even to think this way since I am an Asian woman. I am supposed to be shy, demure, not sexually assertive. The stereotype of the Asian woman didn't encourage me to talk about my sexual excitement and desires; I have been taught since birth to say what other people expect and want to hear.

Growing up as an Asian woman I found no encouragement to explore my femininity or sexuality. Not only were my parents conservative, but with seven older brothers and sisters living in a cramped home in Seoul, Korea, I had no privacy and thus no sex life beyond a few unfulfilling moments of sexual self-exploration stolen while in the shower or hiding under the sheet. Even though my family eventually emigrated to Los Angeles, I was expected to live at home until I married.

I have not always been a feminine, hot, sexy Asian woman. I had to learn to be feminine, hot, and sexy. The movie *9½ Weeks* awakened my sexuality. It was February 1986. I was twenty-three years old and practically a virgin; I had never had an orgasm with intercourse. In a dark, sold-out theater in Hollywood, I got wet watching the movie. I dreamed of having a sexual relationship with a man, even if only for nine or ten weeks. I wrote in my journal, "The most motivation to live is to have an orgasm for one full minute. All that I do is preparing and struggling to get the ultimate pleasure, an orgasm." I used several scenes from the movie for inspiration during my infrequent and secretive (because I still lived with my family) masturbation sessions.

Despite the movie, I didn't know for many years what a sexual animal I was. I was always a bit of a rebel, so while still unmarried I ultimately moved out of my family home in the Koreatown section of Los Angeles. But I did not make that move until I was thirty-four (!), when I got a full-time teaching job. I was much too late in learning about my physical body and what pleasured it. Once I had the privacy of my own apartment, however, I found that my animal sexual instincts were quite strong. Later, I had to learn to express my sexual self to my boyfriend (who became my husband). Then, in order to write this book, I had to find a way to fully express myself to you, showing you the real me with no holding back, no political correctness, no self-censorship. Some of my language choices and descriptions of sexual situations in this book are as frank and raw as I think necessary to convey my thoughts to you. I hope you'll find that they are natural choices in the context of the subjects being discussed.

In my twenties and early thirties, I had a bit of a feminist attitude: I'm a nice, good person, I thought, and it doesn't matter what I *look* like; I'll find a man on my terms. But the truth was that I was desperate to be able to *think* I was in a relationship with a man, any man. Being without a man was unthinkable for me, leaving me no meaningful life. Again and again I chased after men. I was not shy or quiet. I approached men, initiated contact, and pursued them. I carried too many extra pounds on my four-foot-nine-inch frame. I paid little attention to my makeup, hair, or clothes. I had always thought that my best quality was my niceness, and that once I had forced myself on a man he would discount my obesity, my lack of fashion sense, my acne, and my tomboyish ways. If the American Geisha is a perfect example of "being" receptive, I was the perfect example of "doing" things wrongly. I often bought meals, gifts, and even flowers for men; I pushed myself on each of them. A man would fall in love with my niceness, marry me, and we'd start a family, I fantasized.

Of course, I was totally wrong, and this fantasy of mine never came true because roughly twenty men ran from me, avoided me, showed no interest in me whatsoever. I was willing to put up with anything just to avoid being alone. But none of those men ever cared to get close enough to discover my niceness.

Why I Wrote This Book

At age thirty-five I had a bad breakup with my boyfriend of five years. I finally decided to do something about my situation: unmarried, with no prospects of marriage. So I did. I bought just about any and every dating book I could find. I felt that I didn't have time for much trial and error. I needed some spectacular ideas that would work for my personality, my character, and my Asian cultural ways, ideas that would be comfortable for me to use in pursuit of the right man for me. Out of my experience, the books I read, and the research I did, I created my own approach—what I now call my Geisha Consciousness—to find the best man for me, including eventually losing forty pounds. It would take me the next twenty-one months to meet, date, and marry the man I call my "Good Man," the right man for me. I was slowed along the way by many mistakes. My own Geisha Consciousness developed very gradually.

I wrote this book because I wanted to save other women from the mistakes I made and the lost time I suffered. (I don't want women to have to endure the loneliness, unhappiness, and ugly-duckling stage I went through.) After I married, my girlfriends asked my advice on how to find and attract men and how to identify a "Good Man" among those they met and dated. My girlfriends' need for suggestions led me to think about other women: Couldn't *all* women adapt my Asian Geisha secrets while searching for their Good Men? If I had taken advantage of Asian Geisha ways and had become what I now think of as the first American Geisha, couldn't I help *all* American women to develop a Geisha Consciousness, to develop their beauty and femininity? Couldn't I help any American woman become an American Geisha, a new, powerful, and feminine type of woman in search of the right man for her?

The Beginnings of an Idea

Arthur Golden's 1997 book, *Memoirs of a Geisha,* and the 2005 movie it inspired, teased non-Asian women, making them curious about the beauty secrets and powerfully attractive qualities of geisha, of Japanese women, and perhaps of Asian women in general.

Many Japanese-inspired fashion and beauty products were introduced immediately before the movie reached the theaters. Coach offered a Japanese silk-and-mink kimono hobo bag. Cole Haan featured stiletto boots covered in antique Japanese silk. Banana Republic launched a limited-edition holiday collection inspired by the movie's wardrobe, including a silk floral kimono sash-tie top, a quilted geisha bag, an Asian-style tassel necklace, and a satin kimono dress. Facial and body creams featured cherry-blossom-themed packaging and the same image of the movie's star, Zhang Ziyi, that graced billboards, newspaper ads, and even the cover of a special edition of the book.

In late 2005 American women heard a lot about the Japanese geisha. Yet what relevance could the geisha have for American women beyond a book to read, a movie to watch, and some expensive boots to wear? My investigation into the history of the geisha in both Japan and Korea, combined with my research with over four hundred Asian and American single women and men, convinced me that the Asian Geisha (my term for the blending of the Japanese *geisha* and the Korean *kisaeng*) offers many lessons for American women who want to be married, soon, to their Good Men. The golden age of the Japanese geisha and her attitude toward men dates from 1841, when she was accorded by law the status of "entertainer" or "artist." I have adapted Asian Geisha practices somewhat to fit twenty-first-century Western/American culture while continuing to emphasize the geisha's performance or entertainment skills. In particular, I have upheld the concept of the Asian Geisha as embodying the archetypes of beauty and femininity.

Why You Should Read and Use This Book

I believe you are a feminine, hot, and sexy lady, *right now*. But perhaps, like me, you have not been in touch with or expressed this side of yourself very well. You can, though. We all can be American Geisha. All of us have the potential to be beautiful, feminine lovers and wives who will attract, satisfy, and keep our men in love with us forever. The goal of this book is not just to help you become more feminine and sexy in order to get married, but to go beyond that and help you both keep your husband happy and be a happy wife, forever.

In Japan the experienced geisha pairs with a geisha in training through a ritual that bonds them as Older Sister and Younger Sister. As the first American Geisha I want to bond to you as your Older Sister, dear reader and Younger Sister, and help you learn the ways of the Asian Geisha so that you, too, may become an American Geisha.

I will explore the feminine and sexy secrets of the East from what I call a Geisha Consciousness, an awareness of how important a woman's beauty, femininity, and sexuality are to a happy relationship with her man. I will give you honest and clear advice that I have learned from my research and study and also from my husband, who has helped me to be a more feminine woman. As you read and practice the secrets of this book, you will become, more and more, an American Geisha, an incredibly feminine, sexy woman who will attract, satisfy, and keep her Good Man.

I used many of these lessons myself to pursue love and marriage. I will highlight my successes and also tell you how I went wrong, hoping to keep you from repeating my mistakes on your road to love and marriage.

For single women who want to be married soon, this book represents an important goal, showing the way to the destination you aim for when you start looking for a man: love, marriage, and sexual surrender to your partner. I will share Asian Geisha secrets that can help you reach marriage to your Good Man within the next twelve to eighteen months. (Why take twenty-one months, like I did?)

For married women, this book is your checklist and reminder of how to add a spark of caring and passion to your marriage. Your husband has wined you and dined you and spoiled you because he didn't want to lose you, and because you helped him to decide that he wanted to marry you. Now it's time to spoil him by giving him your most beautiful and feminine American Geisha self. He has committed to fathering your children and to providing income and emotional support to the family the two of you have created. As your Good Man's loving wife, you will now reward him for life with your total commitment to his happiness, sexual and otherwise.

Politically Correct? Not!

I need to say just a little about political correctness. I sometimes speak in this book in a politically *incorrect* way. I have to be honest, frank, even outrageous with you. I can't try to cover my little ass, saying politically correct things so that no one gets upset. I won't be politically correct, but I promise I'll be *practically* correct, advising you to do what works, what is practical, what makes you more beautiful, sexy, and feminine in order to attract and keep your own masculine Good Man. If I do deviate at times from what society suggests is proper, please do not be offended. Rather, try to suspend judgment of whether my words are "correct" or "incorrect," and examine them in terms of whether they are empowering and helpful in pursuing love and marriage with a Good Man.

I hope, too, that all of my Younger Sisters can momentarily relax your feminist guard a bit and listen to your Older Sister's advice and suggestions with an open mind. I hope that in the end, dear Younger Sister, you will see me as *both* a feminist and a feminine woman; I see no reason for having to choose one or the other. Do you? Can't we be feminine feminists? I can. I believe you can, too, dear Younger Sister.

In this book I will deal approvingly with some Asian Geisha stereotypes if I find them helpful. I'll tell you to be thin not fat, pretty not plain, accepting not confrontational. I'll tell you that in relationships men are simple, visual, sexual beings who will do most anything to make you happy when you make them sexually happy.

Even as I happily accept some useful stereotypes of Asian Geisha and other women, if other stereotypes are not useful, I'll encourage you to ignore or change them in your thinking or actions, as I did. Still, some strict feminists will question my outrageous ideas and feminine and sexy tips for attracting men. An American Geisha is not a strict feminist, except in the world of work and career. In the world of love and romance, I suggest that you shift your perspective to that of a *feminine-ist,* a woman who values, loves, and wants to operate out of her femininity.

In a sense, in your work world you must insist upon being treated like "one of the boys," treated equally with the men. However, in your personal world, you do *not* want to be one of the boys. You want to be very *different* from the boys, very feminine in contrast to their masculinity. Be a *feminist* while making a living, and be a *feminine-ist* while making (or seeking) love. As a feminist, compete fairly with men at work; then, come home and attract men to you as a feminine-ist.

As much as some feminists may have problems with me, I have no problems with feminists. All women need the feminist backbone that can allow them to be feminine without being weak or passive, to be nice without being taken advantage of. The American Geisha develops within herself a comfortable balance between feminist and feminine-ist qualities.

"Too Submissive"?

In circulating chapters of my manuscript for feedback, I sometimes was told that my advice made a woman too "submissive" to a man or to men generally. I can *understand* that point of view, but I *disagree* with it. My advice simply accepts the truth about (most) men:

- Men are visual and love beauty in a woman.
- Men are sexual and love sexiness in a woman.
- Men are masculine and love femininity in a woman.

By making yourself beautiful, sexy, and feminine for potential Good Men, you are only "being submissive" or "surrendering" to the realities of men and women and to what can help you attract those Good Men to you. I don't want to be too defensive here. In fact, rather than making you submissive, I believe my advice *empowers* you. Beauty and a sexy femininity tend to give a woman confidence, more power, and greater control in finding love and marriage with a Good Man. Isn't this obvious to you? Don't you sense how beauty and a sexy femininity are your allies, your friends in seeking the happiness of love and marriage to a Good Man?

Go on a Fun and Exciting—Even Outrageous—Journey

Part One of the book gets you started on your journey to love and marriage. It deals with developing your Geisha Consciousness (Chapter 1), exploring your sexual, sensual body (Chapter 2), and increasing the beauty and femininity of your Geisha Attractiveness (Chapter 3). In Part Two I discuss sex secrets, such as always crediting him for your orgasm (Chapter 4), finding your G-spot and female ejaculating (Chapter 5), and worshipping his manhood (Chapter 6). With Part Three I help you to plan your quest for love and marriage by defining your Good Man (Chapter 7), developing your marriage plan (Chapter 8), and getting to your most beautiful weight (Chapter 9). Finally, in Part Four you'll find lots of ideas for dating and for after you are married, including how to get to the engagement-ring stage (Chapter 10), when to say, "I could only do *that* for my husband" (Chapter 11), recognizing that love is more than just good sex (Chapter 12), and keeping your love and marriage your highest priority (Chapter 13).

The whole process of finding and marrying a man and then keeping your marriage alive and happy should be a fun experience. (Why do people think that it is so difficult to find a man, not just any man, but Mr. Right, your Prince Charming, a near-perfect-for-you man, a husband, your Good Man?) Do you want to have an enjoyable and exciting time or a difficult time finding your man? It depends on your attitude, your Geisha Consciousness. I suggest we go on a fun and exciting—even outrageous—journey to attract appropriate men and then to choose and to keep your one Good Man for life. The journey begins right here, as you read this page. Get ready to be outrageous, my Younger Sister! Relax. Loosen your bra straps and get ready for some feminine, hot, sexy Asian secrets for finding, marrying, and keeping your Good Man. Get ready to become an American Geisha.

Part One

★

First Steps in Becoming an American Geisha

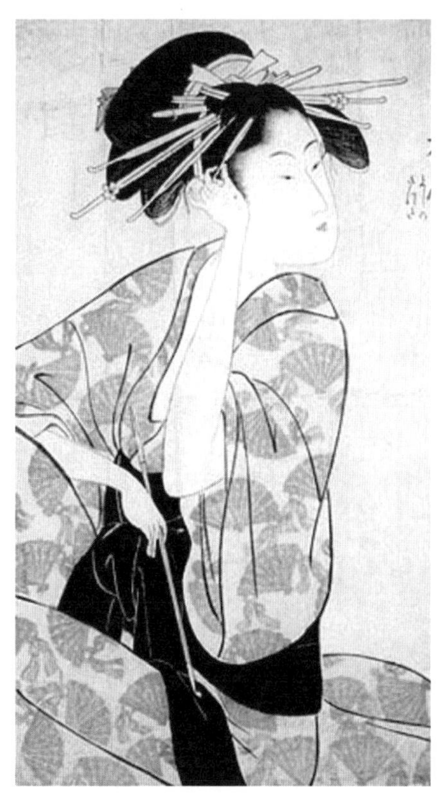

CHAPTER 1

Develop Your Geisha Consciousness

In her pursuit of sexuality, love, and marriage, can any woman become an American Geisha by using the powers, secrets, and lessons of the Japanese *geisha* and Korean *kisaeng?* What is it about the secrets of a feminine, sexy American Geisha that is so incredible that you should learn them in order to attract and to marry the right man for you, what I call your "Good Man"? How can you become an American Geisha? Why would men be attracted to an American Geisha and want to take her to bed or to the altar? You'll find the answers to those questions in this book. I do have some important secrets and lessons for you from the world of the Asian Geisha and from my own experiences, especially if you want to be married, and soon.

What Is Geisha Consciousness?

In the professional development of the Asian Geisha, the younger geisha in training or apprentice geisha (known as a *maiko*) is taken under the wing of a more experienced *onesan* in a solemn ceremony that confers on them the familial relationship of Older Sister and Younger Sister. The Younger Sister *maiko* even changes her name to incorporate part of the name of her Older Sister *onesan*. While I do not suggest you take a part of my name as your own, I do want us to have an Older Sister–Younger Sister relationship as you read this book and practice the actions that will help you to be married soon, specifically within twelve to eighteen months, to your choice of a Good Man for you. Let your Older Sister American Geisha share her experience and research to help her Younger Sister become a happy, successful American Geisha.

The first feminine, sexy American Geisha secret I want to share with you is that we women need to have a particular attitude toward our men, similar to the attitude of the Asian Geisha toward her men.

We have to spend a moment talking about perhaps the greatest of all American Geisha sex secrets: The feminine, sexy woman, Asian or non-Asian, has the mentality of a geisha. Although the modern conception of the geisha goes back to mid-nineteenth-century Japan, the geisha is to this day an important part of Japanese culture. The relatively few women who are willing to spend the many years of training required to be a geisha become quite learned in the ways of ladylike, classy behavior and entertainment in the living room. They are also well schooled in the feminine ways of pleasing their men in the bedroom (as opposed to simply mastering a variety of sex positions). I reveal to you here both the feminine and sexy secrets of the bedchamber, the mysteries of physical love that will bond your Good Man to you, and those of outside the bedchamber, which will first attract him to you. But even more fundamental to understanding the geisha than knowing her talents in bed or out is an understanding of her way of looking at the male-female relationship, what I call her Geisha Consciousness. The Asian Geisha has mastered the art of using all aspects of her femininity to attract, satisfy, and keep her men happy with her so that they will take advantage of her services again in the future. She is, as it were, building a satisfied clientele and a successful long-term business.

Men Are Inspired by Your Femininity, Your "Yin"

The key to using your Geisha Consciousness is to realize the power and strength that lie within your femininity as expressed in a geishalike manner. As I've mentioned, your man is a simple, predictable human being in relationships. He is not nearly so complicated as are we women. (Even Sigmund Freud couldn't figure out what women want, but it's easy to figure out what men want, isn't it? Well, isn't it?)

The Asian Geisha knows that her man is a simple creature who cannot be *legislated* into treating her well, but rather must be *inspired* by her personality, kindness, beauty, and sexy femininity to treat her well, both sexually and in all other aspects of relationship, love, and marriage.

Your Geisha Consciousness realizes that your man is a lover of the yin and yang differences that, in ancient China, Taoists believed attracted men and women to one another. That is, your man wants to experience and enjoy your great femininity (your yin) in order to boost both his own ego and your sense of his great masculinity (his yang). This attraction between opposites, so well understood by the Asian Geisha, is the key to your attracting, satisfying, and keeping your man for a lifetime. As an American Geisha, you will embody to him the differences and contrasts between your feminine and his masculine, and you will encourage and support him in the expression of his embodiment of the masculine. The geisha (Asian or American) knows that there is much truth in the old saying "Opposites attract." Your differences from a man are what attract him to you. Your female characteristics exert a strong pull on his male characteristics as he experiences a gravitational attraction to you and all you represent of the feminine.

The Asian Geisha knows that she should do all she can to make her man feel more masculine, more of a man. She knows that she wants to be as feminine to him as she can be. The American Geisha, too, loves the contrast—the yin and yang—of the differences between men and women, and knows that a man is highly attracted to a feminine woman who encourages his own strong sense of masculinity. Doesn't *any* woman want to be more feminine and have her man feel more masculine? Isn't there just a little moistness forming in your vagina as you think about the passion generated when your great femininity comes together sexually and emotionally with the confident masculinity you've inspired in your man?

The Asian Geisha is seen in Japan and in Korea as being the embodiment of femininity, an old-fashioned femininity, very much a prefeminism femininity. This is what I believe men seek out in the Asian Geisha: the appreciation she demonstrates for the power of her own femininity in relationship with men, what I call her Geisha Femininity. The Asian Geisha has been compared to a doll by both those who approve and those who disapprove of the geisha tradition. The white face of the *maiko,* or apprentice geisha, gives her a porcelain, doll-like quality, simple and even childlike in appearance. This is not a sophisticated femininity but a rather exaggerated femininity, especially when combined with the *maiko*'s very colorful and feminine kimono and shoes. It is this obvious femininity that the male clients want when they ask that a *maiko* join them at an event or party. They do not seek a more subtle femininity (such as that of the unpainted, full geisha in her simpler kimono) so much as they do the more obvious, youthful femininity of the *maiko,* who generally outnumber the Older Sister geisha in attendance at these functions.

As an American Geisha and a feminine-ist, you want to display to appropriate men your obvious femininity, setting yourself apart from other women who appear to be less feminine than you. Your Good Man is more likely to be attracted to a beautiful and clearly feminine woman than to another woman who seems less so. The secret for both the Asian Geisha and the American Geisha is to display her femininity in a *classy* manner. If either the *maiko* or the American Geisha is seen as unclassy, she loses the respect (and attention) of the very men she wishes to attract.

"Feminine Woman" Fever

The attraction to Asian women can be so strong that some Western men develop an Asian fetish, known as "yellow fever," which causes an increase in male body temperature and heart rate triggered by some combination of the woman's great femininity and mysterious Asian looks. I believe it is not so much the Asian appearance of such a woman but rather her overwhelming femininity that attracts men to her. When Western or American women use the Asian Geisha's ways to express their own femininity, they will attract men by triggering "black fever," "brown fever," or "white fever" in them. I believe it is fundamentally a "*feminine* woman fever" that our potential Good Men suffer: the strong, compelling desire to find a truly feminine woman—no matter her ethnicity—to complement their own sense of masculinity. Here's what a few men told me in my research:

> "A feminine woman is someone who is herself, first and foremost. She's intelligent; can use her eyes to smile, connect, and carry on a conversation; and has poise." — Mike

> "I think femininity is related to simply the way we as men perceive the woman we are looking at. She has to be slim, sensual, sexy, and exotic. Femininity is also in the way women carry themselves." — Carlos

> "A woman who is nice-looking and has a very nice body, who knows how to use it and how to dress and act can achieve her wildest dreams and pleasures." — Greg

> "First, of course, her look, dress, makeup. Second, her way of talking and looking at people. And her smile." — Keith

> "The thing that makes her sexy is how she holds and presents herself. If she moves and acts in a subtle and flirtatious way, then a man is likely to

be very stimulated by her. If she wears clothing that just slightly reveals some of her body and gives a hint of what she hides underneath, then I would consider that to be very sexy." — George

These men, it seems to me, are responding to how feminine a women *looks:* her nice body, her makeup, her smile, her way of talking, how she moves and presents herself, her poise. Of course, beauty and femininity come in all sizes, as does sexiness. Your Geisha Consciousness recognizes the full range of attractiveness in taller or smaller women, younger or older women, thinner or curvier women, stay-at-home moms or corporate-oriented career women. Geisha Consciousness is available to *all* women. We can all be more beautiful, feminine, and sexy, no matter what unique combination of body type, psychology, and lifestyle choices we embody. The woman (you!) who goes out into the dating world must represent her true self, who she really is, or else nothing will work out very well in the long run. Your Geisha Consciousness knows that you must be your authentic self, who you really are at your core, as you apply your Older Sister's advice in terms of your appearance, your beauty, your fashion style, your sexuality, and your behavior toward men. In fact, your cool, assured, and comfortable relationship with your real self is, *in itself,* very feminine and sexy to the Good Men that you'll meet.

Femininity Defined

I need to spend a little time here, early in our journey, to clarify an American Geisha's definition of femininity. In reading this book so far, you have encountered some version of the word "feminine" seventy-four times already. So let's see exactly what that wonderful word means.

For the American Geisha, "feminine" most represents those qualities in women that are in contrast to the very *different* qualities that we refer to in men as "masculine." The human body is, first and foremost, the *physical* manifestation of either yin (female) or yang (male) energies. Men's bodies are angular, built for speed and strength. They are designed to be aggressive, to hunt and pursue, to protect and provide. The hormone testosterone that courses so strongly through a man's blood vessels provides him with a chemistry that differs greatly from a woman's (though we women, too, have very small amounts of testosterone in our systems). Men are yang.

Women's bodies are softer, contoured to comfort and nurture. We are yin. The hormone estrogen dominates our blood chemistry (although men have a very small amount of estrogen in their bodies). In her 2006 book, *The Female Brain,* neuropsychiatrist Louann Brizendine, M.D., takes these differences beyond the bloodstream. In an interview she said, "I know it's not politically correct to say this.... But I believe that women actually perceive the world differently than men. If women attend to those differences, they can make better decisions about how to manage their lives."[1] The American Geisha knows intuitively that the brains of men and women sense the world—including relationships—differently. Isn't this *psychological* difference obvious to you, dear Younger Sister?

The Asian Geisha recognizes the power of her receptivity and her nurturing tranquility. She develops these qualities into mysteriousness and elusiveness, which inspire in her male clients a sense of chase. In doing this, she taps into the fundamental vein of masculinity: a testosterone-charged aggression. She makes men hunt her. The Asian Geisha is very aware of her yin versus the male yang.

So, too, should you, dear Younger Sister, embrace your yin. By making yourself explicitly aware of your *natural* femininity, you will appeal to men's *natural* masculinity, and you will facilitate and encourage the bringing together of these two powerful physical and psychological energies into a wonderful relationship with your Good Man.

A Quick but Important Caution

You can only present yourself in this totally feminine way when you are dealing with what I call a "Good Man." In Chapter 7, I define the basic characteristics that make a man a "Good Man" as opposed to an inappropriate (though not necessarily "bad") man for you either to date or to marry. In your Geisha Consciousness you are too soft, open, trusting, and vulnerable to be in relationship with anyone who is not a Good Man, because a nongood man could take advantage of you, hurt you, and waste your precious time. When you are dealing with a Good Man, however, your femininity operates in safety as it supports his protective masculine expression.

Until you determine that a man is, in fact, a Good Man, keep your feminist guard on alert; only interact with him more fully from your feminine-ist self after he has proven himself to you to be a Good Man. (If you are particularly curious about the definition of a Good Man, perhaps because you feel you've too often gotten involved with men who are not right for you, you may want to skip ahead and read Chapter 7, "Define Your 'Good Man,' " before learning more in this chapter about developing your Geisha Consciousness.)

Finding a Good Man will be so good for you, as it has been for me. You will get to express your deepest feminine qualities to your Good Man, who, responding to your powerful femaleness, will bring his inspired masculinity to your love relationship and marriage.

Embrace Your Geisha Consciousness

As your Older Sister I will lead you into many areas of your femininity. In Chapter 3, I suggest many ways to increase the expression of your beauty and femininity. I want you to embrace the Asian Geisha attitude, to internalize the geisha mindset, to focus with total enthusiasm and sincerity on bringing to your love life a Geisha Consciousness.

All of my suggestions or secrets will support you in being the essence of femaleness to him so you can support him in being the essence of maleness to you. Whew! I'm getting hot just thinking about the chemistry of such feminine and masculine essences coming together in a love relationship between two good people, you as a Good Woman and your Good Man. I want you to get hot and excited, too. Let your imagination run wild; see yourself forever in love with and married to a wonderful, masculine man who brings out your deepest feminine qualities. Imagine the intensity and joy not just of the sex, but also of living life together with this fantastic man who thinks of you as the most feminine, fantastic woman he's ever known.

No Manipulation: Tell Your Good Man What You Are Doing

Let your Good Man know that you are learning about and developing your Geisha Consciousness especially for him, so that you can make him happier and happier, both in bed and out. Let him know that his goodness to you and his expression of his caring masculinity inspire you to learn the mysterious ways of the Asian Geisha, so that you can bring him even more of the feminine secrets of love.

Always give him full credit for inspiring you to your greater Geisha Consciousness. Let him know that it is not just your natural way to be so hot and sexy and feminine, but also the influence of finally finding a truly Good Man that has brought out all of your latent femininity and sexuality. Only with him are you so free, so trusting, so feminine, so sexual, so uninhibited.

Tell him, and then show him, that the deeper and more committed your relationship becomes, the more you will feel a growing commitment to his happiness, both sexual and otherwise. If you are already in a committed relationship (but not yet engaged or married), it is especially important to let this Good Man know that many more and greater pleasures lie ahead as your relationship deepens into greater commitment. If you are already married, let your Good Man husband know that your love for him, and his for you, inspire you to do all you can to make him as happy as possible.

Geisha Consciousness involves no secret manipulation of men, so once you think he may be the Good Man you wish to consider for a long-term relationship and marriage, buy him a fresh copy of this book and encourage him to read it and discuss it with you so that he may see the wonderful, loving, sexual future that your relationship has the potential to offer to the both of you.

Commitment and Sex

You have probably heard the expression "Why should he buy the cow when he's getting the milk for free?" What your Geisha Consciousness knows and will subtly communicate to a man you are having a sexual relationship with, assuming he is a Good Man for you to marry, is that while the two of you are involved in quasi-committed dating, he is experiencing and receiving from you only the watery, low-fat, but somewhat tasty milk that the American Geisha makes available when her heart is not fully committed. With his greater commitment to you (and yours to him), which begins with your engagement (with a ring and a set wedding date), he receives from you an increased focus on his happiness, sexual and otherwise.

To carry the cow analogy forward, you will now provide his eager lips with the luscious taste of the cream from the top of the milk. Happily for him, your Geisha Consciousness holds still greater pleasures in store for him when you two are fully committed and settled into marriage. Then he will find that the cream he thought incredible has been surpassed by deliciously sweet, rich butter.

In a word, your American Geisha expression of femininity and sexuality increases as you savor your Good Man's deepening commitment to you. As he rewards you with greater commitment, you are inspired to bring to him more and more of the feminine love secrets that make up your Geisha Consciousness. Without marriage, he doesn't get the butter and cream of your femininity, the best and most joyously enthusiastic sex and intimacy that you can possibly offer him. It is not that you manipulate him with more and better sex as you both become more committed, but rather that he inspires you with his love and commitment to share with him even more of your incredible femininity. Let him know this.

The Biggest Difference Between an American Geisha and an Asian Geisha

You offer more of your heart and soul and sexuality to your Good Man as you grow more deeply attached to and in love with him, and as he loves and commits to you more deeply. This is a distinct difference, the largest of differences, between the Asian Geisha and you, the American Geisha. For the Asian Geisha, her interactions with men (which most often do not involve sex) are her profession; also, of course, she interacts with many men, with the goal of treating them all well. The Asian Geisha does not marry (and if she does, she often must retire as a geisha) and does not believe in romantic love between only two people, as this is not conducive to building her geisha-services business.

You, of course, wish ultimately to identify just one Good Man, fall mutually in love, and marry. As an American Geisha, you wish to take the Asian Geisha's professional secrets and apply them to your *personal* life. The Asian Geisha entices and satisfies many men, but none may marry her (though they may become madly passionate to do so). On the other hand, you, the American Geisha, ultimately wish to entice and to satisfy and, yes, to marry only *one* man, your Good Man. You are sisters, the Asian Geisha and the American Geisha, although your ultimate goals (that is, a good business and a good marriage, respectively) are very different. I feel that I am a sister to you both, to the Asian Geisha and to the American Geisha. For you, I want to be your Older Sister, helping you to find the success I have found, while my knowledge and study of Asian Geisha make me feel like the Younger Sister to those practitioners of these ancient secret arts. Let your Older Sister help you attract, satisfy, and keep the Good Man that you want to marry. Let your Older Sister help you to become an American Geisha.

Reminders While Reading This Book

I suggest you *do* and *remember* the following things while reading this book:

- Decide that you want to be more beautiful and feminine, and commit yourself to that goal.
- Accept me as your Older Sister trainer.
- See yourself as my Younger Sister American Geisha in training.
- Start to make plans to be married within twelve to eighteen months (unless you feel you need longer that that, in which case you should choose a time frame you are comfortable with).
- Be inspired by the concept of Geisha Femininity.
- Develop your Geisha Consciousness over time.
- Be more conscious of your expression of sexuality and femininity.
- Believe in the yin/yang of opposites attracting.

- Be careful and sure that you are involved with a Good Man.
- Increase your sexy femininity with a sense of class.
- Know that a Good Woman doesn't manipulate men.
- Save the cream and the butter (and even the milk!) for a committed Good Man.
- Be happy and enthusiastic about the process of finding your way to a greater sexuality, love, and marriage.

Your Geisha Consciousness has begun to develop. You are moving toward becoming an American Geisha.

CHAPTER NOTE

1. *Newsweek* magazine, July 31, 2006, 46–47.

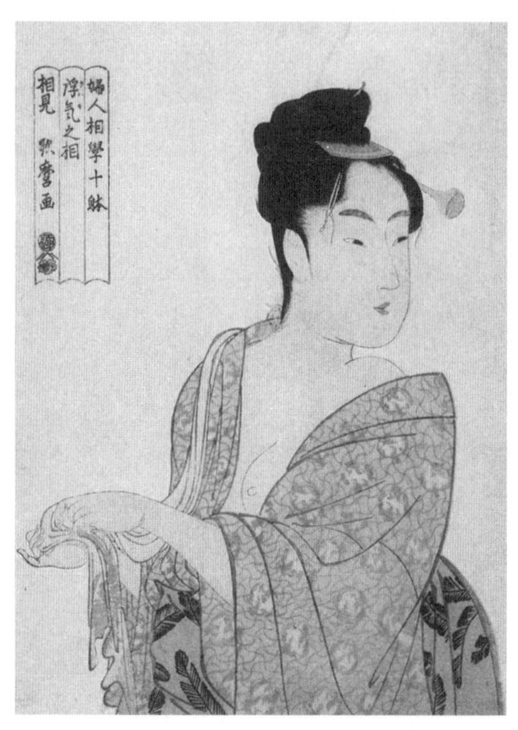

CHAPTER 2

Teach Your Animal Body to Be Sexy and Feminine

As I said in the Introduction, despite the fact that the movie *9½ Weeks* awakened my sexuality when I was twenty-three, I still didn't know for many years what a really hot, sexual animal I was. I never got fully in touch with how much latent sexuality I had, or how much I loved to fuck and to be fucked. I missed so many years of pleasure. I don't want you to miss any years or months, not even days. I want you to start *today* to get in touch with your body and your sexuality. Now, dear Younger Sister, now. I had to learn to be feminine and sexy in 1997 at age thirty-four, when I first started living alone, away from my family. I was much too late in learning about my physical body and what pleasured it. And I didn't masturbate to get to know myself, as I will suggest that you do. I masturbated because my two longer-term boyfriends, Scott and Neil (names changed for their privacy), wouldn't fuck me.

The Story of Scott

In the summer of 1986 I met Scott while on a trip to Europe. During the two weeks we spent together in the Greek Islands, Scott accused me of having a too-tight vagina and suggested that I undergo surgery. Back home from the trip, I spent half a year putting one finger and then two fingers in my vaginal hole to stretch it so that Scott could get inside me when we saw each other again that winter. Scott lived in Scotland and I was in Los Angeles, more than five thousand miles apart. (This story is my husband's favorite. He laughs hard in disbelief that a man would ever complain about a small, tight vagina.)

I kept up a long-distance relationship with Scott for three years although I knew that our sex life was not good at all. (I didn't know that Scott, only forty-four, had an erectile dysfunction problem.) To me sex was just a tiny part of our relationship. Respecting and missing him were more valuable to me than sexual intercourse. You could say I was young and naïve. Or stupid.

In almost three years, Scott and I saw each other for only three vacations together. When I finally ended the relationship, I quickly (without taking any quiet time to consider what I had done wrong with Scott or what I wanted out of my next relationship) got involved for short periods of time with other inappropriate men, including one who was married.

The Story of Neil

In 1992 I met Neil in Los Angeles. Neil's ever-present depression and my constant pressure to keep a dying relationship alive meant we had almost no intercourse after the first year of our five-year relationship. I insisted on maintaining the relationship although Neil never even acknowledged that we were boyfriend and girlfriend, only "friends." I often gave Neil a hand job or a blow job, and he'd come. Then he'd say to me, "Why don't you use the vibrator?"—meaning by myself. He wouldn't participate at all, despite having just received a very enthusiastic, energetic—if unskilled—blow job from a very hot woman. I wound up frustrated and at times begging him for sex, which he chose to dispense to me at about the rate (and I'm generous here) of once a month or less; and, sorry, no cunnilingus, ever! My vagina ached for his tongue but never knew that touch, though I gave him countless blow jobs. Not fair, Neil.

In the last of our three years of dating before Neil left for Korea to teach English, we had sex about once every three months. While Neil hardly ever fucked *me,* I found in his suitcase just before he left for Korea about fifty condoms and three books on how to make love to a woman. My heart felt so sad. I'm still sad when I think of how I allowed myself so many years with these two men who failed to fulfill my animal sexuality. So many years with Wrong Men.

Your Self-Love Sessions: Self-Examination and Masturbation

I believe that all women are, by definition, sexual animals as one important part of their total selves. This chapter will help you to get in touch with and express that lustful animal nature in you. You'll experience the power of your sexuality. And later you will learn that the combination of your femininity and your sexuality is a vital aspect of love and marriage with a Good Man. You'll see how your femininity and sexuality can be so important in attracting, satisfying, and keeping your Good Man. Unlike me, you will be fully aware of your sexual potential and will pursue relationships only with Good Men who, as an important part of your total relationship, will *want* to satisfy your sexuality, and *often.*

Your journey to discovering and experiencing your beauty, femininity, and sexuality while searching for love and marriage with a Good Man starts *today,* as you read right now. Hold this book with one hand and keep reading. With the other hand, stroke over or under your clothes the area of your clitoris and vagina. Go ahead. Do it now, just for a moment, just to get started today on your journey. (Of course, you want privacy, so listen for approaching roommates, spouse, or kids.)

Feel a bit outrageous as you play with yourself. To be hot and sexy, it is necessary to have many sexual experiences—both alone and with a Good Man—and to reach orgasm frequently; it is necessary to be able to fully explore your animal, sexual nature and desires. Of course, all human beings *are* sexual animals, just like all other animals. We are also a "higher" animal. I'm afraid we emphasize the "higher" a bit too much and tend to live our lives out of our brains, out of our "higher" intelligence. We don't get into our bodies often enough—into our "lower," but so sexy, selves.

Begin this sexual exploration *now,* today, before you begin your search for your man. Begin *now* if you are dating. Even if you are currently in a monogamous relationship or marriage, right *now* you want to begin actively to explore your deepest, most animal sexual needs. It is important to begin to explore your femininity and sexuality so that you can become comfortable (and proud!) of your vagina and your physical, animal sexual desires. If your journey to marriage is to be a twelve- to eighteen-month undertaking, then the first day you stroke your vagina and use your mirror to examine it is Day One of that journey.

To have an environment conducive to exploring your sexuality, you must have your own room outside of your parents' home. Don't wait until you are thirty-four, as I did, to move out on your own. Do it *now,* with roommates if necessary. Doing so may be expensive, but you must have the privacy of your own bedroom in order to explore your sexuality. You Younger Sisters who are married or in long-term committed relationships also need to plan some time when your partner is not home and your children are reliably asleep or away from home. Lock the bedroom door.

I want you to find privacy so that you can explore your own sexual needs and desires. Even if you are already a woman of some sexual experience and satisfaction, this hot, sexy American Geisha recommends that you find private time to become even *more* sexually intimate with yourself, before you begin your search for your man. (Of course, you'll also continue to masturbate while you date, and even after you are married!)

Items for Your Self-Love Sessions

To begin, you'll need to purchase these three items for your self-love sessions:

- One, two, or three battery-operated vibrators
- A two-sided mirror with handle
- Baby oil, unscented mineral oil, petroleum jelly, or such water-based lubricants as Astroglide or K-Y Jelly

This is all the equipment that you absolutely need. You may already own the mirror and lubricant. Either now or later, once you are familiar with your vagina and its sexual responsiveness and desires, consider adding the following items to further expand your explorations and pleasures:

- Incense and candles, because your sense of smell can be so powerfully erotic
- Sexy music, to help you set the mood
- Silk sheets, because they feel so sensual
- Sexy silk lingerie, because it feels so good on you and you look so sexy wearing it
- Perfume, because it makes you feel so feminine
- Soft-core guy-girl or girl-girl videos, with story lines as well as sex
- Sexy literature and magazines, both stories and photos
- Sexy fine art (paintings, photographs, sculpture), to add an element of class
- A plug-in vibrator, such as the Hitachi Magic Wand

- Hard-core guy-girl videos, without stories—just hard-core fucking and sucking
- Other sexy toys, such as handcuffs, ropes, masks, clothes, and dildos, to fulfill some of your sex fantasies

As a feminine and sexy woman, you must get to know your vagina (or "cunt," a perfectly acceptable alternative word for the female sex organs, though I won't often use it in this book) both visually and sensually. Let me put it this way: You cannot be a feminine, sexy woman if you do not know your vagina intimately... and proudly!

A few words about terminology: So as not to offend some readers, I use "vagina," rather than the four- or five-letter slang alternatives, to refer to the female genitalia. Even though the vagina is technically only the interior portion of a woman's genitalia (specifically the canal leading to the cervix), for the sake of convenience I usually use it in this book to refer to the entire female genital area. The precise word for the exterior female genitalia is "vulva." A man pees with his penis, but he makes love with his cock. I use the word "cock" in this book; you should use it, too. And, sometimes, to "have intercourse" or "make love" will suffice; at other times "fuck" will seem most appropriate.

Shave Your Beautiful Vagina

Su Nu, one of three female sex advisors to the legendary Chinese Yellow Emperor, Huang Ti (who took the throne in 2678 b.c.), advised him that "a desirable woman has a tender, pliable temperament, with a liquid voice, black and silky hair, soft muscles, and small bones. She is neither too tall nor too short, neither too large nor too small. Her vulva is high up front; her mons is hairless; and she is rich in fluids. She is between twenty-five [and] thirty. While copulating, her fluids flow abundantly, and her body trembles helplessly and is covered with perspiration."[1] I hardly think the Yellow Emperor's sex adviser was right to limit the age range of a desirable woman to between twenty-five and thirty. Eighteen to eighty-five seems more reflective of 2006. Nor do I think any woman is too tall or too short to be totally feminine and beautiful. What I do like is the advice that a desirable woman's mons (or mound of Venus) should be "hairless." In Asia, such a woman is known as a White Tigress, her hairlessness compared to a rare tigress without stripes, and is thought to be very feminine and frankly sexual.

To appreciate the absolute beauty and sexy feminine quality of your vagina, please shave carefully and totally, all the way back to and around your vaginal opening. If you like, you may leave a short, wispy, thin, well-trimmed vertical strip of pubic hair directly below the navel and above the clitoris that indicates to a man that you carefully cultivate the garden of your vagina and clitoris. Maintain this garden; once you are in a relationship, keep this soft, beautiful skin naked by shaving *daily*. Both you and he will feel more sexual with your inner and outer vulval lips, clitoris, and vaginal entrance fully revealed and oh so beautiful and attractive. The almost babylike softness and smoothness of your shaved vaginal area will feel so good both to you and to his fingers, tongue, and cock.

To put it simply, the sexy American Geisha secret that I reveal to you here is that your vaginal area and clitoris are too beautiful to hide from either yourself or your man, and that the presence of pubic hair beyond just a wisp is not sexy and feminine to most men.

Men are hairier than women; they often have quite hairy bodies. Heavy body hair is a masculine, yang, trait, not a feminine, yin, trait. The American Geisha knows that her now nearly hairless body is, generally, in stark contrast to the man's larger, hairier body. Opposites do attract. Your Good Man will love this difference and will feel himself to be a more masculine man, large and relatively hairy, while seeing you as a nearly hairless, feminine woman. My vagina gets a little damp just thinking of how all the elements of my femininity make my man more masculine, both to himself and to me. His cock probably twitches just a little bit toward greater hardness just thinking of his feminine, fully shaved woman.

Another of the Yellow Emperor's female sex experts, known as the Woman Plain, said that the woman who meets the standard has "slender limbs, delicate tissues, soft flesh, elegant texture, skin pure white and pale, finger joints slender and hollow, ears and eyes elevated.... She has no body hair, her body is as smooth as silk, and her pubic region is as soft as grease. If you practice the Way with this kind of woman you won't get tired all night, and as the husband you will be benefited as a consequence."[2] Again, ignore the counsel about skin color, and notice the advice about a lack of body hair, smooth skin, and the genital area being "as soft as grease."

The Asian Geisha is taught over a period of many years the various secrets of how to excite, lure, and entice men. In a word, how to *attract* men. As an American Geisha you too must learn, but much more quickly, how to be a feminine, sexy, sexual woman. (Other elements of the Asian Geisha's training, such as the art of conversation, dance, song, music, and even the elaborate tea service, are, of course, beyond the scope of this book.)

To repeat myself (because the lesson is so important), the Asian Geisha knows that she should do all she can to make her man feel more masculine, more of a man. She knows that she wants to be as feminine to him as she can be. The American Geisha, too, loves the contrast: the female yin and the male yang, the stark differences between men and women. She knows that her Good Man is highly attracted to a feminine woman who encourages his strong sense of masculinity. Men want to feel quite masculine. And men are attracted to a woman who both *sees* and *appreciates* their masculinity, and who supports them in increasing their feeling of masculinity. The Asian Geisha's secret is that she knows that a man's ego and sense of himself depend in large measure on both his feeling masculine and being seen as such by his woman. The Asian Geisha strokes the man's ego in many ways, both to satisfy him at the moment and to encourage him to purchase her business services again in the future. You, the American Geisha, support and stroke your Good Man's ego by making him feel like "more of a man" whenever you interact with him. Your physically naked vagina and your proud naked-vagina attitude awaken in him a greater sense of masculinity in contrast to your visually obvious femininity. Of course, your goal is not future business, but future marriage. Or a perpetually hot, loving marriage—perhaps sexually reinvigorated by your newly naked White Tigress vagina—if you have already found and married your Good Man.

Looking at Your Vagina

You have vibrator, lube, and handheld mirror. And you have shaved your vaginal area naked. Now it's time to acquaint yourself with your genitals. For the very first session you'll want bright lights, so that you can use the mirror's two sides (close-up and extra close-up) to see in magnified detail your vaginal and anal areas, often hidden in that visually inaccessible place down there between your thighs.

Let's hear again from the Woman Plain: "The slit between her thighs is high, there is no hair on her pubic region, and her emission fluid is abundant.... During intercourse, her emission fluid overflows and her body moves and shakes. She can't control herself; perspiration flows in all directions, and she behaves in accord with the man."[3] As you examine yourself, or just at the thought of examining yourself, your vaginal walls may start to secrete their own lubricant. If you are wet, dip your finger lightly into your vagina, bring the wetness out, and spread it slowly over your vulval lips, the entrance to your vagina, and your clitoris. If you are not wet (enough) naturally, use a little of the artificial lubricant to make touching and rubbing comfortable, but not so much that you lose the stimulation caused by the friction of your fingers as they caress, glide, stroke, and pinch their way across, around, and into the various parts of that hidden landscape high up between your thighs.

This very first examination, conducted in bright light, is meant to provide you with an education, an informed awareness of the beautiful, sexy organs that reside just out of your sight. Use your mirror well, especially the extra-close-up side, and admire the beauty of your vagina. You may want to prolong this first bright-light viewing (and touching), or repeat it several times, until you have a pretty good idea of what's down there, how good it can feel, and how beautiful and erotic it is, naked and perhaps somewhat swollen with blood, engorged from your growing sexual excitement.

You may not know that each vagina is as different physically as one fingerprint or one snowflake from another. Let a shiver of passion pass through you as you slowly contemplate, in great detail, the unique vagina that your eyes behold, a gorgeous vagina like no other, ultimately a sexy and beautiful gift for your Good Man.

If you aren't already in a relationship, know that someday a lucky Good Man will gain access to your vaginal entrance. And he will praise his good fortune to be in such a lovely woman's beautiful vagina, to have been worthy to be granted entrance into such an intimate, privileged, almost sacred part of you. For now, though, you are just looking and touching, alone, getting familiar with this feminine center of your sexuality.

This book is about attracting, satisfying, and keeping a Good Man; it is not a medical textbook, so I will not detract from our focus on the feminine and sexual by going into too much anatomical detail, just the basics at this point. Later, in Chapter 5, when we discuss your G-spot (yes, it exists in *every* woman!) and the phenomenon of female ejaculation (yes, you can be a "shooter"), we'll get into somewhat more necessary detail.

For now, focus your attention on your outer vulval lips (the labia majora), and on the clitoris and its hood, which are one of the centers of your sexual excitement. They are located where the outer vulval lips meet, toward your belly button. Poking out from between the labia majora are the labia minora, your inner vulval lips, the thin, butterfly-like, and very sensitive folds of skin that often swell and fill quite noticeably during sexual stimulation. Of course, you'll also want to give proper attention, externally as well as internally, to your vaginal opening. And locate with the tip of your index finger the very important urethral opening (where you pee), located between the clitoris and the vaginal opening. Finally, trace lightly toward the rear over the smooth, sensitive skin of the perineum, located back toward the anal opening (between the anus and the vaginal opening). **(Caution:** If you explore inside the anus, be sure to wash your hands and vibrator thoroughly before using either in the vaginal area, in order to avoid introducing even microscopic fecal material from the rectum into the vagina or urethral opening.)

Once you have examined and touched your vaginal area enough to feel fully aware of and comfortable with all of its physical aspects, it is time to begin exploring your vagina's sexual responses and desires. If looking at your genitals involved some real work in maneuvering the mirror while trying to get Hollywood-style lighting to fall on your vagina just where you needed it in order to see well, then masturbation will be the play part of your exploration. Perhaps switch to soft lights or semidarkness. Candles? Incense? Sexy lingerie? Position your body on the bed so that it is much more relaxed and natural. Start with just your fingers, using one or both hands to hold, stroke, pinch, tease, separate, and penetrate as your desire leads you. Let yourself respond to your own touch in a natural, uninhibited way. (You are in your own bedroom, aren't you? Door locked!) Let yourself moan, groan, pant, cry out, scream as your vagina's and clitoris's excitement grows, perhaps to orgasm, with your fingers' movements.

Stroke your thighs, pinch your nipples, squeeze your breasts. Suck vaginal juice off of your fingers with your mouth, lick it off and taste it on your tongue. Use the vaginal juice on your fingers like a lipstick, to sensuously paint your nipples or facial lips or to apply lubrication just to the tip of your clitoris, as you lightly circle the clitoris with just the very tip of your finger. Luxuriate in the wonderful, sensual feelings you bring to your animal body. Don't let your mind inhibit your enjoyment of your beautiful, feminine body. Experiment with different amounts of pressure on your clitoris, as well as with direct stimulation of the clitoris and indirect stimulation of it through the hood that covers it when it is unstimulated (before it starts to swell and expose itself). Run your fingers gently over your belly, your thighs, the undersides of your breasts, wherever your touch feels good. (Using lubrication on these body parts will increase your pleasure.)

My vaginal walls are sweating lubrication even as I write this, beginning to fill my vagina with the wetness of sexual excitement. I'm breathing just a little hard. And, hey, I haven't even suggested yet that you turn on your vibrator. I will, though, for no matter how turned on you are just from manual (finger) stimulation, an American Geisha knows that the vibrator is an indispensable sexual asset in masturbation (as well as an invaluable partner while having sex with her Good Man).

If you haven't used your vibrator up to this point, turn it on now. I have several, including one I like so much that I have a nickname for it: the Horse. You may have used one earlier, during the examination phase. Or you may have started your masturbation with the vibrator rather than with your fingers. All of that is just fine, and fun. Use your vibrator (or more than one type of vibrator) at *any* time, whenever you feel like it. If it feels good, do it. With a man, or without. (Maybe *not* while driving—but at a traffic light...?)

I've suggested that you buy several vibrators, in part because some provide a stronger and some a lesser vibration; some are variable speed; some are larger or smaller; some are louder or quieter; some feel more like plastic or rubber or skin; some even have removable attachments. Find the ones that turn you on, that make you feel like a hot, sexy American Geisha, happy and *proud* to be finding out how your fingers and vibrators can excite you. Discover whether your excitement is greater with fingers (one? two? three? four?!!) or vibrator penetrating your vagina, or with a nonpenetrative focus on your clitoris and vaginal lips. Or one vibrator in your vagina, another against your clitoris. Again, whatever feels good, excites you, and makes you come. And come again. And again (why stop?).

Be playful. Smile at your outrageousness. Enjoy a quick moment of embarrassment at how loudly you moaned or screamed when you came hard with the vibrator pressed firmly against your clit (clitoris) as your wet finger touched and stroked that so-sensitive, blood-engorged pleasure site.

Women who possess Geisha Consciousness know that sexual pleasure is good, healthy, and, yes, fun. The American Geisha knows that only when she can *comfortably* please herself sexually will she be able to bring to her Good Man the greatest of sexual pleasure, both for him and for herself. As you examine your vagina and masturbate to orgasm, you are moving along the path toward becoming a very hot, sexy, sexual American Geisha.

CHAPTER NOTES

1. Valentin Chu, *The Yin-Yang Butterfly: Ancient Chinese Sexual Secrets for Western Lovers* (New York: Tarcher/Putnam, 1994), 88.
2. Howard Levy and Akira Ishihara, *The Tao of Sex* (Lower Lake, CA: Integral Publishing, 1989), 130.
3. Levy and Ishihara, 129–130.

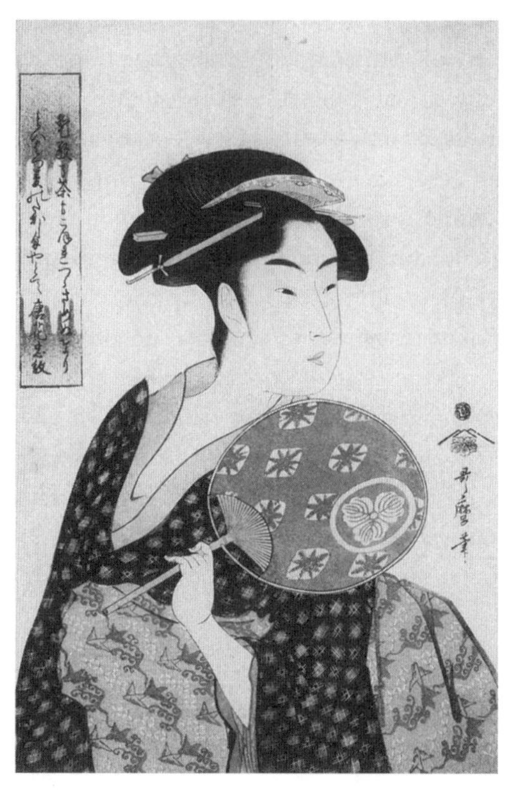

CHAPTER 3

Geisha Attractiveness: Beauty and Sexy Femininity

> She had a pale, refined, pretty face, softly oval, with a sensuous mouth which curved into a provocative smile, and almond eyes brought out with just a hint of makeup. She was lovely in a feminine way rather than intimidatingly beautiful.
>
> But it was less her appearance than some indefinable presence that set her apart. She was poised, confident, funny, and charming. She would, I imagined, be any man's perfect woman—sexy yet motherly. To me, as a woman, she had another face. We talked girl to girl, though she still gently, so that I hardly noticed, made sure that my glass was full and that I had everything I wanted. I was perfectly taken care of, in fact.
>
> — *Leslie Downer, author of* Women of the Pleasure Quarters, *writes of her meeting with an off-duty, Western-dressed geisha, Shuko*[1]

It was a rainy day in 1985. At the L.A. City College library I saw a student I liked. We had often passed each other on campus and said hi. I walked over to him and asked if he could give me a ride home. He said to me, almost angrily, "Are you insane? Why do you think that I am interested in you? You don't act like a woman. Why would I care to talk to you?" I was shocked. In that moment I felt like a total loser. I was insulted and hurt. What else could be a worse way to hurt a woman than to say, essentially, "You are not a woman"? But that was the truth in men's eyes. I was not seen or noticed as a woman. My niceness didn't impress men. Inside, I knew I was a nice woman, but my outside appearance made men not even think of me as a woman. This was true because I wasn't dressing and acting like a woman, and I was heavy and unattractive—not pretty, not sexy, and not feminine.

Unfortunately, even after that humiliating encounter in the library at age twenty-two, I didn't decide that it was time for me do something about my lack of beauty, sexiness, and femininity until I was thirty-five, a full thirteen years later. I didn't realize right away that I had to do something to help myself. I had been hurting myself by believing it didn't matter how attractive I was. Even that rude slap in the face in the library, and much more humiliation with other men, somehow didn't wake me up to the fact that my lack of beauty and sexy femininity was keeping me from the relationship success I so wanted.

Furthermore, it took me many years to learn that most men want to be the hunter, not the hunted. After much (negative) personal experience and a lot of reading, I finally realized I had to *attract* a Good Man to me, not stalk and ambush him, which had been my approach.

I can't believe how out of touch I was with the reality of men, especially to have bought into the *un*truth that only what was inside (my kind personality) should be enough to find love and marriage with a Good Man. As you develop yourself in your pursuit of love and marriage, Younger Sister, I want you to avoid being called an "ugly duckling," as one man yelled at me as he retreated from my assault. Or, "not really a woman," as another described me to my face. I want you to attract Good Men to you, not to have to fend off nasty men's nasty comments.

I should have known that instead of using all my energy to pursue a man, I needed to become attractive to a man and to let him pursue *me*. When I started to do something about my weight, my makeup and clothes, my acne, and my unfeminine ways, I noticed that men were paying me more attention.

Even if you are married or already in a committed relationship, Younger Sister, you still want to increase your Geisha Attractiveness. Similarly, the American Geisha who is currently seeking a husband should continue to work on her Geisha Attractiveness even after she marries, because the ultimate objective is not simply to attract a Good Man and to marry him; the objective is to have a long, loving, happy, sexy marriage. We all need that spark of passion in our marriages, and your ongoing attention to your beauty and femininity (your Geisha Attractiveness) will ignite his ongoing hot desire for you.

The Power of Geisha Femininity

The Asian Geisha represents the epitome of femininity; as I've discussed, her whole professional life can be fairly summarized, I think, as a maximizing of her sexy femininity so that her male clients can maximize their own sense of masculinity in their relationships with her. This is what they pay for in hiring geisha services: to feel good about themselves as masculine men. This example of the fundamental femininity of the Asian Geisha is the greatest lesson that she can teach us as American Geisha: To attract, satisfy, and keep your Good Man, be so beautiful, sexy, and feminine that you bring out the best aspects of his masculinity. Make him feel good about himself as a man. Do that, and he'll never leave you.

The stereotype of the Asian Geisha is a woman who is thin, with ironed-straight black hair, flawless skin, and an exotically different face. This stereotype reflects the truth that men notice a woman's body type, her weight, her hair, her skin, and her face. Men take note of all these things because they are very visual creatures; they are attracted to what looks good, whether it is a car, a house, a painting, a meal, or a woman.

The Asian Geisha does not fight against this stereotype; she does not demand that men be attracted to her for her other, less superficial qualities. Instead, the Asian Geisha focuses on making herself as visually attractive, sexy, and feminine as she can, knowing that this is what *first* attracts a man's attention: the sight of a beautiful, sexy, feminine woman.

During the second half of World War II the geisha districts were closed and many geisha worked in factories. Mineko Iwasaki, one of the most celebrated of Japan's geisha and a primary source for Arthur Golden's novel *Memoirs of a Geisha*, quoted her Auntie Oima's recollection of that time:

> Even though it was wartime, those of us who lived in Gion Kobu [one of the geisha districts of Kyoto] competed with each other over who had the most beautiful silk work clothes [cut out of their kimonos]. We attached collars to our necklines, and braided our hair neatly in two long braids, and wore sharp white headbands. We still wanted to feel feminine. We became famous for lining up, heads held high, to go to work in the [munitions] factory.[2]

The Asian Geisha knows that the stereotype of Asian beauty is a positive one that can be useful to her. She understands that as she adheres to this stereotype, clients tend to be *attracted* to her, and her success as a geisha grows. In turn, the American Geisha understands that she can adapt all of these Asian Geisha characteristics to Westernized concepts of beauty, sexiness, femininity, and other elements of a woman's attractiveness to men.

Again, from Mineko Iwasaki:

> A maiko in full costume closely approximates the Japanese ideal of feminine beauty.
> She has the classic looks of a Heian princess, as though she might have stepped out of an eleventh-century scroll painting. Her face is a perfect oval. Her skin is white and flawless, her hair black as a raven's wing. Her brows are half moons, her mouth a delicate rosebud. Her neck is long and sensuous, her figure gently rounded.[3]

The Western or American man is attracted to (or at least notices and appreciates) any fit, well-groomed woman who plays up her uniquely beautiful characteristics and expresses her inherent femininity. You can be any age, race, height, or ethnicity, and if you have enhanced your Geisha Attractiveness you will draw the very focused attention of many men. Most men's eyes will lock onto the image of a beautiful, feminine woman, and many will risk straining their necks as they swivel their heads just to keep that image in view for only a few more seconds. It has taken me quite a while to understand that men are so appreciative of *any* woman's beauty and sexy femininity. When we are beautiful, even men who merely see us in passing may celebrate their good fortune at being in just the right place at just the right time to have observed us. Just a few moments of a pleasing image on his eyeballs can make a man's day. Men are so visual. And so simple. And we women can all be so attractive to them.

My husband helped me to learn this about men when he called me to the TV to have me watch a commercial that he said was definitely aimed at a male audience. I don't even remember what the advertised product was. But as I recall, the commercial showed a well-dressed businessman of about thirty-five walking along a New York sidewalk on his way to work. He drops some papers on the sidewalk and they blow around a bit. As he bends to recover them, a passing taxi splashes him with rainwater from the gutter. Now standing with an exasperated look on his face and damp papers in his hand, he notices a limo pass by slowly, and he catches a glimpse through the lowered window of a beautiful, feminine woman sitting alone in the backseat. They make eye contact. As her driver continues down the avenue, the man—his whole being changed by those few seconds—smiles broadly toward the camera and says, "Sweet!"

Again, Younger Sister, men are so simple and so visual. And they love our feminine beauty so much.

The Asian Geisha works, first, on the beauty of her total body, literally from head to foot. The naked skin of the ankle above her tiny white socks in her wooden shoes is seen by men as quite sexy because she shows so little naked skin. Second, of course, she also works on the beauty of her clothes. Many kimonos cost fifty thousand dollars or more. Third and fourth, she knows that part of her visual presentation to men is how she presents herself as *sexy* and *feminine.*

The Asian Geisha never lets her clients or potential clients see her when she is not at her most beautiful and feminine. Very few men actually live or work in the Asian Geisha areas, arriving there only in the evening. By 6:00 P.M. the geisha have transformed themselves into the stunning women that their clients expect to see in the teahouses and throughout the geisha district.

The Asian Geisha works consciously at always becoming *more* beautiful, *more* sexy, and *more* feminine, even if only by implementing the tiniest of changes. She makes enhancing her appearance and mannerisms a high priority so that she may continue to be thought of as attractive by her male clients and thus remain in demand for her companionship services. Since she is in the business of being a geisha, we can look at her efforts as similar to those of an entrepreneur wanting to make a conscious effort to maintain and to improve the quality of her product, which is herself, so as to maintain her clients' satisfaction and their loyalty to her.

If she rests on her laurels and fails to maintain and improve her attractiveness, perhaps a younger, prettier apprentice geisha will steal her clients and also attract other gentlemen who might have been the older geisha's new clients. The world of the Asian Geisha is extremely competitive, and beauty and a sexy femininity (as well as entertainment and conversational skills) are critically important to each geisha's success.

You know, don't you, dear Younger Sister, that the world of the American Geisha is also extremely competitive, especially when you desire love and marriage with a (relatively rare) Good Man. I needed help to compete, to build my beauty, and to develop my femininity. I'll bet you might be able to use some help, too. Be ready to invest in your beauty and femininity by doing what is necessary to compete for a Good Man. As my readers who are already married know, even after the wedding music has faded, you continue to have competition, not necessarily from other women, but from the inattention that relationships can suffer. Continue to compete strongly by staying focused on your relationship, *and* by remaining both feminine and beautiful throughout your marriage.

What Makes a Woman Sexy and Feminine?

Can *any* of us (you, dear Younger Sister American Geisha, or me) be as beautiful as a model? Perhaps yes. Perhaps no. But this is my point: Can *all* of us be *more* beautiful, sexy, and feminine tomorrow than we are today? Answer that one with me, please, by saying a confident, "Yes, I can be more attractive tomorrow than I am today. I just need to make it a high priority in my life to be more beautiful, sexy, and feminine every day."

As part of my research, I asked both men and women what makes a woman feminine and sexy. Here are some of their responses:

"She is receptive to a man's suggestions and plans."

"She has a way of carrying herself."

"She drips with sexuality."

"She smells good, looks good, and sounds good."

"She is appreciative of whatever I do."

"She has a loving personality."

"It's her way of talking to you or looking at you."

"It's her smile."

"She uses her eyes to connect to you."

"She shows her emotions."

"She has poise."

"She laughs freely and loudly and enjoys life."

"She satisfies her man's fantasies."

"She accepts me for who I am."

"She doesn't take life too seriously."

"She respects her man."

"She sees me as her hero."

"She makes me feel like a man."

"She's a little bit playful."

"She is confident in her beauty."

"She's kind."

"She is not confrontational."

"She is positive about herself."

"She is beautiful and exciting to look at."

"She is a ferocious feline in bed."

"She tells me what she likes [sexually]."

"She screams [during sex]."

"She gets excited [sexually]."

"She never pushes me away [sexually]."

"She never uses sex for power."

"She is gentle and graceful."

"She is shy and naïve outside; inside, she has a huge sexual desire."

"She is sexual, sensual, and erotic."

"It's in the way she carries herself."

"She knows how to dress."

"She knows how to use her body."

"She can use her eyes to smile."

"It's in her way of talking to and looking at people."

"She moves and acts in a subtle and flirtatious way."

"Her clothing slightly reveals some of her body."

"She gives a hint of what lies underneath her clothes."

"She is smolderingly sexy, but always classy, in public."

"She is responsive to the slightest touch."

"She easily reaches multiple orgasms."

"She is extremely oral, both giving and receiving."

"She has highly responsive nipples."

"She has bones like rubber, no matter her age."

"She likes to bite and suck my lower lip."

"The flirting, the teasing, the suggestion."

"She is comfortable being sexually provocative in her appearance."

"She falls in love with me after she has a huge orgasm."

"She is outrageous and sexy on the outside and inside."

"She isn't afraid of public affection."

"She has a voyeuristic side to her."

"She uses a few explicit words in the heat of passion."

"She knows what pleases a man and herself."

When I collected this information, I did not refer at all to geisha. I simply asked respondents what they felt made a woman feminine and sexy. However, if you eliminate all of the explicitly sex-related responses, you'll find upon rereading the list that most of these qualities describe the Asian Geisha in her relationship with her clients.

Likewise, all of these elements of femininity or sexiness give you options and choices in terms of your relationship with your Good Man. You, dear Younger Sister, should consider expressing your feminine, sexy self in some of these ways to the prospective Good Men that come into your life.

Although not all psychologists agree, the research of David M. Buss, as reported in his 1994 book, *The Evolution of Desire: Strategies of Human Mating*, suggests that men are attracted to youthfulness or the look of youthfulness in women and to healthy-looking women. Specific elements of a woman's appearance that were found particularly attractive included full lips; clear, smooth skin; clear eyes; shiny, full hair; good muscle tone; a bouncy, youthful walk; an animated face; and a high energy level. As to body type, men did *not* tend to prefer very thin women, though men were conscious of wanting to obtain a high-status, attractive wife, because such a wife increases a man's standing.

First Be Yourself, Then Be Feminine

I need to pause for a moment and assure you, dear Younger Sister, that I do not suggest that all women become some idealized stereotype of "feminine." Even to have such a thought reminds me of *The Stepford Wives,* which was a novel and a movie in the 1970s and was remade as a movie in 2004. All of the wives in the town of Stepford are incredibly feminine (they do aerobics in high heels, for instance), but also incredibly passive and dominated by their husbands. As two new arrivals to town (Nicole Kidman and Bette Midler in the 2004 version) eventually learn, all the other "wives" are, in fact, robotic clones created at the husbands' request to replace their assertive wives. In contrast, I want your femininity to be an individual, unique expression of who you really are, a femininity that represents you being *more* of yourself, not less, not a homogenized, soulless, robotic slave that devotes yourself totally to your Stepford husband. No Good Woman American Geisha would want to be that type of robotic woman; nor would any truly Good Man want to be with a woman who is not her own real, happy, individual self.

You'll express your femininity differently as a working woman, as a stay-at-home mom, as a student, as an office worker, as a salesperson, as a rock-climber, as a bookstore lover, as a teacher, as a musician, as a clerk, as a jogger, or as a business owner. Your options about how you identify yourself are, of course, almost limitless; so, too, are the ways to express your femininity within these many possible identities. "Be yourself" (*your* self) is good advice. Be *real* to the men (and to anyone else) you meet. Uncover for yourself and then share proudly with the world your best, truest, most womanly self.

As you read this book, continually think about and ask yourself, "What is my real self? Who am I? And how does 'being more feminine' apply to me?" Record some of your thoughts and associated feelings in a journal.

Be Your Most Beautiful, Sexy, and Feminine Self, *Always*

Models and a few other lucky women are born so naturally beautiful that they look good under any circumstances. The rest of us, Asian Geisha or American Geisha, must work to create or enhance our beauty and sexy femininity. Then we must carefully display ourselves so that we always look our best to the men we wish to attract. And, unlike the Asian Geisha, we in the Western world can't wait until after 6:00 P.M. to be beautiful, sexy, and feminine. You need to be at your best and most attractive nearly always, for who can say when you might meet your potential Mr. Right, your Good Man?

In seeking out your Good Man and in the initial stages of your relationship with him, you should accept happily that you will always need to be your most beautiful and feminine self. That's a sexy secret you, as an American Geisha, want to learn from your Asian Geisha sister. You want to attract the attention of lots of appropriate men to allow yourself to have the greatest number to choose from in order to find the one Good Man who is right for you to date or to marry. You need to develop your Geisha Attractiveness, a combination of a beautiful you, the right clothes, sexiness, and femininity. Both the Asian Geisha and the American Geisha initially need to attract men to them. The Asian Geisha's success begins with being able to attract the attention of men who could, after getting to know her better, become her regular clients. So, too, your success as an American Geisha in finding love and marriage begins with attracting men to you, one of whom, after getting to know you better, may become your Good Man and husband.

I want you to consider how important beauty and sexy femininity are to you at this moment in your life, as you seek to find the right man to marry. Or if you are an already-married Younger Sister, think about how boosting these aspects of yourself will enhance both your husband's and your happiness in the marriage. Probably most of us women—single or married—would like to be more beautiful or at least somewhat beautiful. But how many of us are making our beauty one of our highest priorities? I suspect, again, that it may be politically incorrect to say, "I have as a high priority to make myself more beautiful, sexy, and feminine every day." The P.C. police and some feminists might see such a goal as self-absorbed, shallow, and selfish, or, again, as too "submissive" or "surrendering" to what a man likes to see in a woman.

It may be politically incorrect to tell you that a woman should develop these qualities in herself. However, know that a nice, sweet, but unbeautiful, unsexy, and unfeminine woman may spend many lonely, unhappy years being politically correct and unnoticed by most men. I don't want you to go unnoticed as a woman, as I did for so long. It hurts you too much and too deeply. It attacks your very concept of yourself. I know this is true. I experienced it. It hurts me even now as I remember it so many years later.

In the context of finding the right man for you to marry and finding him in as short a time as possible, you must be realistic. The reality is that men, including those who could qualify as your Good Man, are attracted to a beautiful or pretty woman more than they are attracted to a plain woman. I want you to smile to yourself right now, Younger Sister, and say, "I knew that all along." Of course you did. It's just common sense. Everyone knows it. Men are *attracted* to women who are... ready?... *attractive!* If you want him to be motivated by a verb form of the word (to be attracted), then you'd better be motivated by the adjective form of the word (to be attractive). Think with me for just another moment, please. Isn't the masculine type of man you seek (your Good Man) attracted to a sexy and feminine woman more than to a less sexy and unfeminine woman? Again, I hope you agree quickly that the answer to the question is an obvious, "Yes."

If you are already married (or in a long-term monogamous relationship), you want to make your Geisha Attractiveness a presence in your relationship. Your goal is no longer to get a man to make a strong commitment to you, but rather to inspire your man to maintain his strong and passionate commitment to you. I have only common sense to back me up here (no statistics), but wouldn't you just imagine with me that if half of all marriages fail and half don't, those that don't fail probably tend to involve women who make beauty and sexy femininity a *continuing* priority in their relationships?

Look around you every day at all the other women you see. Then ask yourself, "Do many of these women seem to be making it a priority to be beautiful, sexy, and feminine as they live their day-to-day lives?" It seems obvious to me that many do not. Despite the fact that most men require beauty and a sexy femininity from a woman in order to be *attracted* to her in the first place, few women try hard enough.

Do Nothing. Wait. Be Receptive.

Notice that I use the word "attract" rather than "pursue" when I describe the relationship between a feminine woman and a Good Man. The Asian Geisha sets a perfect example of passively, femininely attracting, rather than aggressively pursuing, men in her business life. She *never* calls her customers, *never* initiates getting together, *never* pays for a meal or buys a gift. These are all masculine actions. The Asian Geisha is the absolute embodiment of the spirit of femininity. She readies herself. Then she waits. She has a confidence that she has prepared herself so well that gentlemen will seek out her company, her mere presence in their lives. The Asian Geisha relaxes, waits, and is receptive to the masculine energy that initiates, pursues, hunts, and makes things happen.

As an American Geisha you want to show this relaxed, confident, waiting, receptive attitude, knowing that you have prepared yourself well and that *you need do nothing further*. Simply wait. In a coffee shop, wait to be approached. In a classroom, wait, knowing that you are displaying your beauty and your femininity. At work, wait for the man to initiate conversation. At a dance, smile happily and wait to be approached. Everywhere, wait. On a group hike, in a bar, at a religious gathering, at a party, at a business conference. You are relaxed and confident. You know that you are attractive; you simply wait until your beauty and sexy femininity attract a man.

A caution: When I tell you that you need do nothing more than wait, I do not mean for you to wait at home. You must deliberately do enough to get yourself out into the world and give your attractiveness the opportunity to draw appropriate men to you. In Chapter 10 you'll find lots of ideas about where to go to meet potential Good Men. Once you've gotten away from home, *then* you wait for the man to display his masculinity by approaching the beautiful, sexy, and feminine woman that is you. (Obviously, in a business setting the "sexy" element of your attractiveness is toned down or fully removed.) Once you have prepared yourself by developing your Geisha Attractiveness, and have availed yourself of opportunities to be noticed, then you let the man "do" what is necessary, while your role is simply to "be." Be receptive to the man's actions.

For my married Younger Sisters, you too need to "do" nothing once you've created your most beautiful and sexily feminine self. Your husband will eventually notice, as will other men with whom you interact. When your Good Man husband finds himself even more attracted (or newly reattracted) to his lovely wife, assure him that this change in you is inspired solely by your love for him and your desire to make your marriage more wonderful, even happier and better for both of you. Perhaps show him this book and give your love for him full credit for inspiring you to be your most attractive self. Build your husband up as a man even as you build yourself as a beautiful, feminine woman.

What Do I Mean by "High Priority"?

I want to suggest to you specific, practical things that you can do to become more beautiful, sexy, and feminine. But before doing that, I want to define what I mean when I say that you must make the development of these qualities a high priority.

A high priority is something that you desire strongly, stay aware and conscious of, spend substantial time pursuing, and work hard to accomplish. It is also something in which you may invest significant money.

A simple example will make my point. Imagine that you have a doctor's appointment. It's the doctor's final scheduled appointment for the day, and you absolutely do not want to be late. You will probably remind yourself of the appointment the day before and keep it in mind during much of the actual day. You'll make extra effort to get work and other responsibilities finished early. Despite all of this, if you are still running late you'll gladly pay the money for a taxi instead of taking the bus across town. You do so because you have chosen to make being on time for this appointment a high priority on this particular day. You've decided that other things are not nearly as important as making it to the doctor's office on time.

I am suggesting that finding the right man to marry (your Good Man) and being as beautiful, sexy, and feminine as you can be are so important to you and to your happiness that they should be among your highest priorities. As in the example of the doctor's appointment, any high priority will involve your focusing on it, thinking about it, staying conscious and aware of it. If the ultimate goal is marriage, stay focused on that. If an interim goal is to become more beautiful, sexy, and feminine, stay conscious of that. If you do not stay conscious of these goals, you will almost certainly fail to do what is necessary to achieve them, and thus will almost certainly fail to reach them. To my married Younger Sisters, you must also stay conscious of your specific goals within the marriage; otherwise the reigniting of your relationship is likely to remain just an unfulfilled wish.

Just as you were willing to invest your valuable time and effort toward doing what was necessary to be at the doctor's office on time, so too you will happily spend lots of focused attention on moving toward marriage. You will do the necessary work to accomplish those things that increase your beauty and sexy femininity. You will make the necessary extra effort. And you will spend the necessary time. You do this willingly and enthusiastically because you know that the achievement of these important goals will bring you such happiness.

Much as you were willing to pay extra for a cab to be on time for your doctor, as an American Geisha you are committed to spending your hard-earned income on your highest priorities. Invest your money wisely both in your pursuit of love and marriage and, specifically, in your ever-increasing Geisha Attractiveness.

There is nothing "passive" or "submissive" about you, Younger Sister, as you go about doing the things that need to be done to attract Good Men into your life. You are taking control in order to reach the destiny you have chosen for yourself: to be in love with and married to your Good Man within twelve to eighteen months.

You need to be comfortable with, even proud of, these twin goals—the pursuit of love and marriage *and* of beauty and sexy femininity—so that you exhibit a happy, contagious enthusiasm that will help to attract potential Good Men to you.

Becoming More Beautiful, Sexy, and Feminine in Three Areas

So, to summarize: The hot, sexy American Geisha chooses what she wants (here, beauty, sexy femininity, love, and marriage). Then she pursues her wants with a positive attitude that helps her to attract the right type of men to her: men who are happy and enthusiastic about their own lives.

Now let's look at some suggestions for your hot, sexy self that will help to make you more beautiful and feminine. To start with, let's examine the three areas that the Asian Geisha constantly works to improve: The beauty of your entire body, the beauty of your clothes, and the expression of your sexy femininity.

WORK TO BEAUTIFY YOUR ENTIRE BODY

I want to suggest that no other "beauty factor" is as important in attracting a man's attention as achieving and maintaining your most beautiful weight. You've probably heard the research showing that over 60 percent of Americans are either fat or, worse, obese. This is an incredible fact: Six women out of ten are much too heavy for their beauty or their health. And, of course, still more women are above their best, most beautiful weight. If you are among the 20 or 30 percent of women who are at or near their best or most beautiful weight, then you will have a great advantage (an incredible one!) over those other, say, 70 percent of American women in attracting appropriate men to you.

Being at your best weight is so important that I've devoted all of Chapter 9 to the topic. Don't worry, though. I have a plan for you. Not a diet, but a *plan* to help you reach—and maintain—your most beautiful weight, not an anorexic or skinny weight, but the most comfortable, healthy, and appropriate weight for your body type.

For now, let's just acknowledge how important the right weight—a beautiful weight for you—can be in the eyes of a Good Man, and how important that right weight can be to your own level of confidence and happiness. Be optimistic with me. Because you care so much about love and marriage, beauty and sexy femininity, you will be successful in managing your weight. Then you will be at your strongest and most confident as you pursue love and marriage with your Good Man.

It is appropriate to emphasize weight in developing a hot and sexy American Geisha appearance because extra pounds can have such a specific and significant impact on areas of beauty throughout the body. Notice the correlation between your best weight and a shapely body *generally* with these other *specific* aspects of your beauty:

RELATIONSHIP BETWEEN YOUR BEST WEIGHT AND BEAUTY

Area of body	Beauty revealed when you are at your best weight
Skin	Tight, smooth, soft to the touch, toned
Face	More defined bone structure, smile shows more readily
Breasts	Firmer, more prominent areola and nipples
Eyes	More prominent, distinct
Neck	Narrower, seems longer
Shoulders	Underlying bone structure and muscles revealed, appear toned
Ribs	Bone structure revealed
Waist/stomach	Smaller, flatter shape
Arms	Appear toned, more muscles revealed
Wrists	More delicate
Hands	Smaller, seem longer, thinner
Fingers	Seem longer
Hips	Smaller, no bulges
Thighs	Narrow, no cellulite, possible space between legs up to the vagina
Vaginal area	More visible, isolated from thighs, seems daintier, smaller
Knees	Shapely bone structure revealed
Lower legs	More defined, appear toned, more muscles revealed
Feet	Smaller, not bloated or puffy
Toes	Seem longer

Goodness. Weight seems to impact just about *every* area of your beauty except your hair, teeth, ears, nose, and nails. (And I'm not sure about the tongue.) However, even if you are already at or near your best weight, you may still be able to increase the beauty of these different areas of your body. Let's look again at certain areas of the body and suggest quickly how each might be made more beautiful and sexy:

CHECKLIST OF WAYS TO ENHANCE YOUR APPEARANCE

Hair	Styling (grow out or cut), color, shine, fullness, dandruff control
Skin	Remove or reduce warts, moles, growths, extraneous hair, scars, acne; avoid the sun
Face	Reduce splotchiness, chemical peel or laser resurfacing, clean pores, use makeup (or don't use makeup), sun protection
Ears	Hairstyle to reveal or conceal; earrings, piercings
Eyes	Pluck and reshape brows, makeup (or not) for lids, liner, contact lenses
Lips	Gloss, liner (or not)
Tongue	Scrape or brush
Teeth	Dentistry for shaping and spacing, whiteness, cavities filled
Neck	Jewelry, attention to clothing necklines
Breasts	Remove extraneous hairs, better bra support for display, braless, clothes to reveal or emphasize
Shoulders	Exercise to tone, clothes to reveal or emphasize or flatter
Back	Clothes to reveal or flatter
Ribs	Clothes to reveal or flatter
Waist	Clothes and patterns to emphasize or flatter
Stomach	Exercise to tone, belly button jewelry, clothes to reveal or flatter
Arms	Exercise to tone, clothes to reveal
Wrists	Jewelry to emphasize
Hands	Gloves to protect while working, sun protection
Fingers	Rings

(cont'd.)

CHECKLIST OF WAYS TO ENHANCE YOUR APPEARANCE

Fingernails	Shaping or lengthening, grooming cuticles, polish
Hips	Clothes to reveal or flatter
Thighs	Exercise to tone, pants and skirts selected to flatter (e.g., tight pants to reveal space between thighs; looser pants for meatier thighs), shorts, short skirts or bathing suits to reveal shapeliness
Butt	Exercise to tone, pants or skirts to flatter, bathing suits or shorts to reveal or flatter
Vagina	Shave to reveal
Knees	Shorts or skirts to reveal
Lower legs	Exercise to tone, high heels to emphasize muscles, boots to flatter
Ankles	Thin gold chain or socks to draw eye, shoes to reveal
Feet	Barefoot, sandals, open-toe shoes to emphasize, pumice for softness
Toes	Toe ring
Toenails	Polish, shaping

Just as weight loss can positively affect beauty in a general way, so can exercise of various sorts affect the beauty of your skin, shoulders, arms, back, breasts, stomach, upper and lower legs, and butt. Of course, you could always undertake invasive surgery for such things as breast augmentation or reduction or liposuction of thighs or stomach. Though you could do this, I will not recommend it. I believe you can use the weight plan in Chapter 9 and some simple, completely noninvasive procedures to increase your beauty without resorting to surgical procedures. Haven't I suggested quite a goodly number of actions you could take that would not involve the surgeon's knife and the anesthesiologist's skills? Over time, accomplishing some—not necessarily all—of these little improvements in your appearance will add up to a big, obvious change in your overall beauty. You can literally spend months and years becoming more beautiful and feminine every day, just a little bit at a time, just a little bit more each day.

There are a very few situations in which I believe a woman might want to consider surgery. Most noses are just fine as they are, but if yours is somehow beyond the rather expansive range of "normal" or has been damaged by injury, consider rhinoplasty to reshape and resize it. Noses are not usually a critical area of beauty, because it is not an element of the face that men usually focus on. I believe that men usually notice the hair, eyes, mouth, and shape of the face before they notice the nose or ears. The ears are a second possible candidate for surgery. But again, only if they are remarkably misshapen (rare) or overly protruding from the head (somewhat more common). As to the breasts, I believe that all shapes and sizes are seen as beautiful by different Good Men according to their preferences. Consider breast-reduction surgery only for overly drooping, pendulous breasts, or overly large breasts that distort the natural beauty of the areola and nipple or that cause back pain or other physical discomfort. I do not believe a woman should *ever* have surgery to enlarge her breasts. Small breasts are not just "fine"; they are beautiful! (My husband says, "Any more than a mouthful is wasted anyway.") If childbirth or other events have left you with a loose, inelastic vagina (and if you are not helped by the Kegel exercises described in Chapter 5), you might want to consider "vaginal rejuvenation" surgery, for both your Good Man's and your own increased sexual-emotional satisfaction. Finally, if the connection between neck and chin is obviously sloped, creating a "weak chin" or "chinless" appearance, it may be a strong candidate for corrective surgery.

I do not recommend that you follow *all* geisha habits of beauty and femininity:

> After finishing at the hairdressers, I went to the barbershop to have my face shaved, a common practice among Japanese women. My face was shaved for the first time by my father after he gave me my first haircut, on the day I turned one year old. I have had it done once a month since then.[4]

One last thought about the beauty of your body before we move on to consideration of your wardrobe. When you do something that increases your physical beauty you often increase a man's perception of your sexiness and femininity at the same time. For instance, if you lose excess weight you'll probably increase your beauty. At the same time, the average man would also probably see you as sexier and more feminine, since a heavy size is generally regarded as unsexy and unfeminine. If you remove unwanted hair from somewhere, chances are that many men would say that you look sexier and more feminine since "hairiness" (except on the head) is considered a masculine trait.

We American Geisha are quite fortunate that as we make ourselves more beautiful, we may also be perceived as sexier and more feminine. I think of it as a womanly "bonus" of sorts. The same is true of your wardrobe: Beautiful clothes can help you to look more feminine and sexy.

WORK TO IMPROVE THE BEAUTY OF YOUR CLOTHES

I was so oblivious to fashion that I should have looked into getting some professional help with my wardrobe selections. What about you? Don't you want to dress with a sense of class, whether you go upscale or middle-class, urban chic or artsy bohemian or sporty fresh? Of course you do. Even when you dress sexily, you don't want to project a low-class image, do you? Do you want your clothes to complement your physical beauty and to have a feminine (and, if appropriate to the setting, a sexy) quality? This can be done on any budget because it has more to do with taste and judgment than it does with the actual cost of the clothes.

Become more fashion conscious. Subscribe to two or three women's magazines that appeal to you, according to your interests, your age, your geographical location (rural or urban), your profession. Be open to the fashion and makeup tips offered, but certainly not a slave to them. Pay attention to the seasonality of fashion. Approach those of your girlfriends who seem most attractive and well put together for help. Ask for some tips and frank critiques of your fashion sense. If you are lucky enough to have a gay male friend, buy him dinner and wine and see if his insights about your clothes and use of eye shadow or lip color could be helpful. If you seek professional help by approaching a cosmetics counter for a makeover, be cautious! I've seen some pretty scary makeup jobs on the very women who offer to teach you what would be flattering on you. (Don't they look in their own mirrors?) Remember, you know yourself best, so don't surrender total control over your look to a stranger who is probably working on commission. Often, less is better. And, of course, the best for you may be no makeup, or just enough so that it *seems* as though you are wearing none.

Unless you have money to burn, I suggest that you consider the resale shops, either a thrift store like Goodwill (where I've found many cute, sexy pieces for three dollars or less) or a more upscale, Beverly Hills–like store that recycles designer apparel at much-reduced prices. Somewhat different in philosophy is the vintage store, where the prices can be fairly high but the merchandise has a more quirky, past-era style to it. Some of the pieces bought in these stores can be improved with scissors, needle, and thread. I like carefully chosen pieces from resale shops for the obvious monetary savings they offer, but also because by wearing them you add a unique flair to your appearance. No one else has exactly the same item as you do, especially after the scissors and needle do their work. I believe that you want to dress differently and better than the average woman, so that you are more noticeable to potential Good Men.

Along with subscriptions to fashion magazines, sign up for a free e-mail subscription to the *New York Times,* where you'll be able to review articles, still shots, and video with commentary regarding the latest fashions. Be inspired by what you see as you put together your own wardrobe.

You'll also buy clothes that are appropriate to your interests and to the socioeconomic environment in which you seek to find your Good Man. Are you outdoorsy (and do you want him to be, too)? Is the theater more your interest? Are you a big-city girl? Small town? Happiest on the farm? Like sports cars or drive a pickup? Wine-tasting events? Art exhibit openings? Love baseball? Prefer tennis at the club? So many possible interests, so many possible men to meet through those interests, and so many wardrobe choices to make based on those (your!) interests.

Whatever the label might say, your goal with your clothes is to highlight your best physical attributes (say, your long, toned, bony back), while masking your weak spots (say, your lower legs). Thus, you might opt for a vertically striped, tight top that hugs your back and ribs, and pair it with full-length, narrow-cut pants. The options are literally countless. Just be sure you know your best physical attributes and dress to attract attention to them. Likewise, be aware of your less beautiful endowments and dress to downplay them. Finally, remember this basic: Dress with a sense of *class.*

WORK TO INCREASE YOUR SEXY FEMININITY

As you think about increasing your sexy femininity, remember that simply by becoming more beautiful and dressing more beautifully, you will tend to encourage men to think of you as more feminine and sexier. Once again, it is that strong connection between beauty, femininity, and sexiness. Fortunately, then, when you work on any *one* of these three aspects of yourself, you receive the bonus of positive change in the other two areas. I do not want you to think of beauty, femininity, and sexiness as three separate and discrete dimensions of yourself. Instead, as many of my research respondents seemed to do, allow yourself to dissolve the boundaries between the three, and see them combined into what I call your Geisha Attractiveness.

I've mentioned that having a sense of class is important. Let me be more specific. Everything you do to attract appropriate Good Men should be done with attention paid to the tasteful and refined image that you want to put forth. A Good Man may or may not have money, a great job, or social standing, but he does have the basic characteristic of dealing with the world in a higher-class way. He operates with honesty, integrity, and kindness. You always want to attract this type of man, and you will do so if you display your beauty, femininity, and sexiness within the context of being a woman with class. Put another way, an American Geisha always engages in the classy behavior of a Good Woman, thereby attracting the appropriate attention of an equally classy Good Man.

You can easily imagine how "class" can be associated with beauty and with feminine behavior. The more difficult association is probably between overt sexiness and class. To begin with, let us remember not to separate beauty, femininity, and sexiness. Instead, let's mix your three-part Geisha Attractiveness with classiness and see how you can set yourself apart from the competition. I'll use just one example from that last long list of what respondents found sexy and feminine: "Her clothing slightly reveals some of her body." When you dress this way, you will be perceived as being sexy, feminine, and beautiful; all three aspects of your Geisha Attractiveness will be on display.

The Asian Geisha must be very careful to do this in a tasteful way or she risks putting off her very class-conscious clients and developing a reputation for inappropriate, unclassy behavior. For you as an American Geisha the situation is similar. You, too, want to attract and satisfy classy men, not so you can build your business but so you can eventually attract the right Good Man to you, fall in love, and marry. Let me suggest a few possible ways to implement "revealing some of your body" with the proper consideration for both your Geisha Attractiveness *and* classy behavior:

- You reveal your best weight and your toned thighs with a black miniskirt (key to classy: not *too* short).
- You wear a traditional business suit to work, with the hem four inches above the knee (key to classy: *not* eight inches above the knee, and custom-tailored to flatter your body).
- You go braless in a classic button-front white shirt (key to classy: not *too* many buttons undone).
- At a party, your neckline plunges practically to your navel (key to classy: nonchalant confidence, yet awareness of maintaining good posture).
- At a party or dance you wear a Wonderbra to enhance your décolletage (key to classy: not too many shirt buttons undone, and your breasts do not look scrunched together under enormous pressure).
- You wear Brazilian-cut, hip-hugging jeans and a cut-off T-shirt (key to classy: the jeans are not so low-cut that your backside looks like that of a plumber fixing the garbage disposal unit under the kitchen sink).

Remember, classiness isn't just about how you dress. You can pick any of the items from the list of what my respondents found feminine and sexy and imagine for yourself how they can come across in a classy (or unclassy) way. Classiness is a concept that each of us, dear Younger Sister, will define somewhat differently, according to our backgrounds and experiences. Whatever your definition of "classy" might be, your Older Sister is suggesting that as you seek to increase your beauty, femininity, and sexiness—in sum, your Geisha Attractiveness—always keep in mind, as the Asian Geisha must, the image you project to prospective Good Men. Remember that the image should always be that of a classy Good Woman.

Finding the Time and Money for Beauty and Sexy Femininity

You must depend on your great desire for sexuality, love, and marriage as your basic motivation to find the time and money to implement your plan to be more beautiful and feminine (much as that same motivation will provide the energy behind your success with your weight and exercise plan; more on that topic in Chapter 9). However, just to stimulate your creativity, below are two short lists of ideas for finding time and money to devote to the further development of your beauty and femininity.

I must anticipate that you may find some of your Older Sister's suggestions a bit bizarre. For instance, I suggest perhaps spending less time with friends and family. I do not mean to devalue either friends (especially your wonderful girlfriends) or family, but only to suggest that sometimes we women can make the mistake of spending inordinate amounts of time hanging out with friends and family when we say we want love and marriage. In effect we are substituting friends or family (or both) for working on ourselves—on increasing our beauty and femininity—and we risk abandoning our highest priority (love and marriage).

As you examine and add to these lists, your Older Sister would simply ask you to consider whether different parts of your current routine really serve you well in pursuing your highest priorities. Keep those activities that give you good feelings, that bring you wholeness, and that make you a confident, relaxed, well-rounded person. See if you can eliminate or cut back on time-wasting activities.

To save time:

- Get a less-demanding job. (I'm serious. If sexuality, love, and marriage to a Good Man are your *highest priority for happiness,* do not let an overly demanding job or career take your focus, time, and energy to the extent that it gets in the way of achieving those goals. Don't let work substitute for love.)
- Spend less time cooking and eating. (Gourmet meals are not a good substitute for love either.)
- Spend less time sleeping (eight hours maximum).

- Spend less time with friends/family.
- Spend less time on dates with inappropriate men. (Spend time with Good Men instead.)
- Spend less time on the phone. (Even unplug the phone at times.)
- Get rid of your cell phone. (Or turn it off frequently, and check messages later.)
- Unplug or (better) sell your TV. (I *know* you watch more than just PBS.)
- Cut back on reading. (*After* you finish this book.)
- Don't seek overtime work.
- Don't work on weekends. (Weekends are for your *personal* life.)
- Say no to unsatisfying or unreasonable requests for your time.

To save or make money:

- Get a smaller, cheaper apartment. (Your Good Man cares *not at all* that you might live in a two-bedroom apartment rather than in a one-bedroom or studio apartment. And he doesn't care what your job is either, even if you do care what his is.)
- Get a smaller, cheaper car. (Just make sure it is reliable and safe.)
- Buy less food.
- Hold a yard sale.
- Use coupons.
- Drink black coffee. (Not a triple-double latte soy frappe with goat's milk.)
- Don't vacation.
- Ask Mom and Dad for (some of) your wedding-expense money up front. (Then pay for your own wedding.)
- Ask for a raise. (It's time!)
- Refinance your home and take some of the equity as cash.

Now that you have saved this time and money, consider *spending* it on your beauty and sexy femininity, as well as on your health.

To spend time and money on your highest priorities:

- Date appropriate men.
- Exercise, take up a sport, join a gym.
- Have skin treatments, get a massage, spend a day at the spa.
- Wake up ten minutes earlier to style your hair (no cost).
- Get a makeup makeover.
- Get a fashion makeover or consultation.
- Go out alone (often).
- Go out with others (sometimes).
- Pick a night to stay in, do your nails (fingers and toes), and apply a mud mask.
- Plan and keep daily charts (no cost; more in Chapter 9).
- Relax (no cost).
- Meditate (no cost).
- Feel and look happy, positive, and optimistic (no cost).
- Participate in singles groups or events.
- Buy accessories and jewelry.
- Spend time every day accessorizing your outfit.
- Buy good clothes.
- Get healthy.
- Sleep enough (no cost).
- Date through the Internet.
- Get your hair styled or colored.
- Soak in a bathtub (no cost).
- Take one tiny step each day toward becoming more beautiful.
- Become more feminine each day (no cost).
- Dance.
- Exfoliate your skin in the shower (no cost).
- Get a pedicure.
- Get a manicure.

- Buy perfume.
- Buy sexy underwear.
- Engage in a hobby.
- Be creative (no cost).
- Experiment with dressing more sexily.
- Masturbate (no cost).
- Buy sex toys and videos.
- Smile (almost always! No cost).
- Reread *Sex Secrets of an American Geisha* (no additional cost).
- Give blood. (You're nice. No cost.)
- Volunteer somewhere (no cost).
- Have a full life. (You're worth it!)

When You Increase Your Options, You Are Making Progress

By my count, in this chapter I have thrown in front of you a total of over one hundred items in five different lists. Perhaps that may seem like too much to deal with. Perhaps you feel overwhelmed because of the sheer number of items. Try to reframe it. I hope you will look at these lists in a positive way. Each list offers so many different things that you might be able to do. Each item offers you an option or a choice:

- Shall I look for a smaller apartment? Or not?
- Shall I put that great dress on my credit card? Or not?
- Shall I start drinking my coffee black to lose weight and to save money? Or not?
- Shall I save time and raise money by selling my TV? Or not?
- Shall I whiten my teeth? Or not?

Options and choices are empowering, dear Younger Sister, because it is *you* who gets to decide which option to choose. You can choose the option that may help you to reach your goal of love and marriage to a Good Man, or another option that doesn't help you to reach that goal. It's your choice. Very empowering.

When you feel like you have no options, things are bound to stay the same, since an option implies change from how things are at the moment. As to my earlier heavy weight, for instance, I believed for the longest time that I had no options. I thought that I had been born with a body structure and shape that were genetically determined and unchangeable. There was nothing I could do about my height (four feet nine inches) or weight. I was stuck with this body type: short and squat. I lied to myself by telling myself this was true. I also thought that weight loss was "just too hard. I can't do it." Both of those beliefs kept me in a rut for years. No options meant no change. I stayed the same: short and squat and powerless to do anything about my situation.

I want you, dear Younger Sister, to realize much more quickly than I did that you *do* have options. In fact, many options, including the more than one hundred items I've suggested in the five lists. This is truly progress, because until you realize that you *have* options, you cannot choose one or more of those options; thus, you cannot change. Options empower you; they put you in control since it is up to you to decide (choose) which option to take (including the option of not changing). The more options you are aware of, the more progress you are making toward fulfillment of your goal, whatever it is.

Many Asian Geisha are quite proud of the independence that the geisha life affords them. The Asian Geisha is a self-sufficient business-woman who makes her own decisions. She depends on no one else. In fact, many people depend on her for their living: the geisha house owner, the tea-house managers, the maids and servants, her male dressers. Even all of the tradespeople in the geisha district depend for their livelihoods on the success of the geisha in attracting and satisfying her clients. Without the Asian Geisha herself, of course, there is no geisha world. She is powerful, aware and proud of her important position in her world.

You, too, as an American Geisha, should be proud of your power to make your own decisions, to choose the options in your life that are right for you. If you want to find a Good Man, fall in love, and get married, you need no one's permission, approval, or agreement. It is *your* decision. You are powerful. Recognize and be proud of that truth. Be happy that you have choices and that you are aware of them. If you are already married to or living with your Good Man, dear Younger Sister, you still have many options open to you as an individual. You can decide to work on your relationship or on your body, for instance. Happily, when you two are already a committed couple, you also have many options open to you, such as jointly working on your relationship or on your bodies.

I want you to reread each of the five lists right now: the correlation between weight and the beauty of different body areas; improving the beauty of each area; saving time; saving money; and spending time and money. As you reread, add to each list whatever further options come to your mind. Remember, with each additional option you think of, you are making progress toward your dual goals of greater beauty and sexy femininity *and* love and marriage to your Good Man. Of course, if you are already in a committed relationship (or if you have children), you may need to add and subtract items from my lists (e.g., a husband or child might rebel at selling the big-screen TV to raise money to buy your hundred-dollar eye cream). Stop reading right here. Go back and add your thoughts to each of those lists, right now. Then come back here and we'll carry on.

You are a Good Woman. You are becoming more beautiful, more feminine, and sexier. And you are doing all of this with a proper sense of class. You are displaying your Geisha Attractiveness to appropriate men. More and more, you are becoming an American Geisha.

CHAPTER NOTES

1. Leslie Downer, *Women of the Pleasure Quarters* (New York: Broadway Books, 2002), 227–228.
2. Mineko Iwasaki, *Geisha: A Life* (New York: Atria Books, 2002), 57–58.
3. Iwasaki, 140.
4. Iwasaki, 140.

Part Two

★

Sex Secrets to Bond Him to You

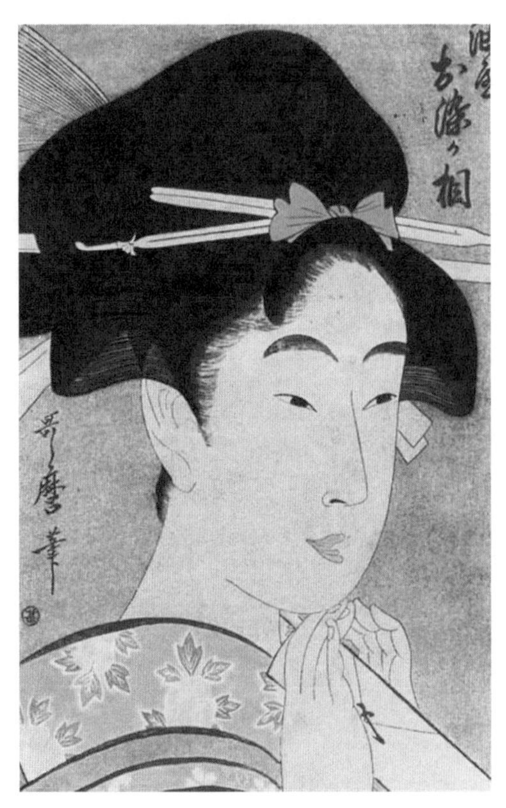

CHAPTER 4

Give Away Credit for Your Orgasm . . . to Him!

Did you know, dear Younger Sister, that men have very fragile egos? Psychologists tell us, but perhaps we women still don't realize, just how fragile a man's ego is. He can feel bad about himself as a man if things go wrong at work, if he performs badly at sports, if he feels disrespected by someone, even if he sees another man with a very beautiful woman.

A man's sense of himself *as a man* is generally much more fragile than a woman's sense of herself *as a woman*. Although men are physically stronger, in the areas of psychology and self-image women are surely the stronger, at least as concerns the fundamental ways men and women feel about themselves in their gender roles. Although a woman can certainly have quite negative psychological reactions to events in her life, it is unlikely that she will often feel fundamentally bad about herself *as a woman*. She may have reactions to different situations that make her feel like a bad friend, an unloving wife, or an uncommitted employee. It is unlikely, though, that she very often thinks to herself, "I'm not much of a woman," or "I feel bad about myself as a woman." Women tend to be secure in this area, not very hard on themselves in evaluating how they are doing as a member of their sex. But imagine, if you have kids, how you would feel if someone attacked your skill or worth *as a mother*. That's how a man feels when he believes that his worth *as a man* is under attack.

I believe that both the Asian Geisha and you, the Younger Sister American Geisha, have a fundamental and firm grasp and psychological certitude of your basic worthiness as a woman. You'll rarely hear a criticism such as, "What kind of a woman are you to do something like that?" Perhaps it is even amusing to think that anyone would try to attack you in that way, for your concept of yourself as a woman is likely a strong one, not easily assaulted.

You might well feel bad if things went wrong at work, but to feel bad about your womanhood for something that went wrong at work is something you probably cannot fathom. After all, you might think, how can the two, work and womanhood, even be considered linked? My other examples of losing at sports and of being disrespected would not cause you, dear Younger Sister, to feel like less of a woman, would they? And if you see another woman with a very handsome man, I am confident that whatever your reaction might be it would not be to put yourself down as a woman.

Part Two of the book is addressed primarily to women who are already in committed, monogamous relationships or who are married, since I recommend that you do not have sex, even with a Good Man, until you commit to a monogamous relationship *and* both test for sexually transmitted diseases. (I'll go into more detail in Chapter 10.) If you are still seeking your Good Man, reading this part of the book now will be valuable in helping you form your Geisha Consciousness. Once you become more intimately involved with a Good Man, you'll want to revisit these chapters to remind yourself how much you can do to make your man feel good about himself and about you.

You Must Be Strong to Pursue Love and Marriage

We women are strong. The Asian Geisha must be confident of herself as a woman as she pursues a livelihood that not all people understand or respect. The American Geisha must have confidence in herself as she pursues love and marriage, since she, too, may be misunderstood by some who don't respect or agree with her steadfast, ambitious pursuit.

Most men, on the other hand, are forever judged (and judge themselves) by whether they act in a *manly* way. (Have you ever thought about anything you've done, Younger Sister, and asked yourself whether you acted "in a *womanly* way"? I doubt it.)

Most men, including your Good Man, feel their manhood threatened by the many ways in which they can be made unsuccessful in their endeavors (such as in work or in sports), or threatened by a loss of control (as in being disrespected). And as for that other man with a beautiful woman, it is in the realm of sex that your Older Sister finds most men's egos to be quite vulnerable. Losses and a lack of control in a man's sex life make him feel bad as a man. Conversely—and here is the good news for the American Geisha who wishes to attract, satisfy, and marry a Good Man—his successes and feelings of being in control in his sex life make him feel good about himself as a man.

Put simply, your Older Sister thinks it comes down to this: A man is expected by others and by himself to perform successfully and to be respected. When he is unable to get the world to grant him these things, he feels like less of a man. Women, in contrast, do not associate successful performance with their concept of themselves as women. A woman doesn't have to *do* anything to feel good as a woman; just *being* is enough for her to feel fine about herself. And while a man feels he has to command respect if he's any kind of a man, a woman is more focused on being cherished or loved. Because women and men are so different in this area, we women may have some difficulty understanding and empathizing with a man about it. "What's the big deal?" we might think when our Good Man seems so devastated and down on himself for making an error that cost his company softball team the game, or when a potential new client (disrespectfully) cancels his sales presentation at the last minute.

Make Your Good Man Feel Like *More* of a Man

I spend so long on this subject because it is so important. For your relationship with your Good Man to be successful, you must *never* make him feel like *less* of a man. You must *always* help him feel like *more* of a man when he is with you.

One of the strongest similarities between the Asian Geisha and the American Geisha is the dedication they share to building up a man's confidence in himself. This is the unspoken, primary motivation men have for employing the services of an Asian Geisha: She makes them feel fantastic. She does this by stroking the man's ego, by devoting herself totally (in the minutes or hours of her service) to making the man (or group of men) the absolute focus of her attention. The client feels incredibly flattered that this beautiful, sexy, feminine, talented, intelligent, confident woman so willingly gives him more focused attention than does any other woman (or person) in his life. Of course, if these men were to examine the situation with a more critical eye, they would probably realize that the geisha is simply providing her skilled services because she is well paid to do so, not because she thinks any particular client is "such a man." The Asian Geisha is a beautiful actress, speaking lines from a script that she has developed for the very purpose of making her client feel good about himself. She knows that a convincing, ego-building performance with her client will likely result in his future business. Even if her performance is simply images and fakery that could not withstand closer scrutiny by her client, he will choose again and again *not* to examine it closely, for he so enjoys the final outcome of their little charade. In her company he feels so funny, so wise, so handsome, so captivating.

Younger Sister American Geisha, it is important that you learn this lesson about men's psyches. Yet it is equally important that you recognize a key difference between yourself and the Asian Geisha. You will build your Good Man's ego and sense of himself as a man through your sincere affection, not through the calculation of customer satisfaction. Let us pause here a moment and consider the idea of the American Geisha's similarity to the Asian Geisha. Over hundreds of years Asian Geisha have prospered by recognizing the great and fundamental need in men to feel good as men, and by providing services to fulfill that need. These services tend to be quite expensive, so the psychological need they fulfill must be quite compelling; otherwise a client might better spend his money on something more tangible. Yet those who employ a geisha's services feel they get good value for their money, and again and again they ask for a particular geisha's attendance at their events and parties.

This psychological need to feel good as a man must be very powerful. Were we able to probe deeply into and even below the consciousness of men who employ geisha services, we might find that their subconscious minds know that it is all smoke and mirrors, all illusion, all a subterfuge, all an unreal image projected by the geisha, who has learned over a long training period how to do what she does so well, to transport her client to an incredible fantasy world where women dedicate their lives to making men feel good about themselves.

You, too, my American Geisha trainee, will dedicate yourself to making your Good Man feel like more of a man whenever he is with you, simply because he is dating or engaged to or married to you. As you might suspect, it is especially in the area of sex that your Good Man can be made to feel so good about himself. It is also where, according to how your sexual relationship works out, he can be made to feel bad about himself as a man. Because a woman's way of looking at sex is so different from her Good Man's way of looking at sex, I believe (and my husband and other men confirm) that it is between difficult and impossible for her to fully comprehend how important it is to a man that he perform well and successfully and be respected by her as a great lover (or, at least, as a quite competent one). Of course, we women do not put such pressure on ourselves to "perform" during sex, and during sex we certainly do not look for "respect," but rather for pleasure, love, cherishing, and caring.

If you, Younger Sister, can come to have this understanding of your Good Man and are sincerely and enthusiastically willing to do all you can to make him feel incredibly good about himself sexually, you will offer to him something that is nearly impossible to find in any other woman. The way to a man's heart is through making him feel better about his cock; the way to a man's heart is through making him feel better about himself as a man. Make him feel good, great, fantastic about the performance of his cock (or fingers or tongue), and you'll make him feel good, great, fantastic as a man. Do this consistently and he'll never leave you.

It is time again for a caution from your Older Sister. I have emphasized in this chapter that you should always make your Good Man feel good about himself as a man. My caution is that you stay conscious of two things as you build up your man's sense of himself: Do this *only* for a Good Man; and do *not* become a doormat by sacrificing yourself and forgetting what *you* need out of the relationship. Both the Asian Geisha and the American Geisha are strong, assertive women who pursue what they need from the relationship, even as they are wonderfully kind and supportive of their Good Men.

Abandon Political Correctness in Bed

I have spent several pages, dear Younger Sister, building my case for making your Good Man feel good about himself as a man, especially as a *sexual* man. Now let me return to the title of this chapter: "Give Away Credit for Your Orgasm... to Him!" I know that we women in the Western world have had to struggle for the right to be acknowledged as both worthy and capable of having frequent, consistent orgasms. Freud tried to make us feel "immature" for having clitoral orgasms; and the G-spot orgasm (see the next chapter) remains relatively unknown to Western women. So, while we are still trying to claim our rightful place in the world of orgasms, how can I recommend that you give away credit for something you've fought for and continue to fight for so mightily, your orgasm? A woman's orgasm almost rises to the level of political rights. Yet I want you to throw credit for your orgasm over to your Good Man, rather than politically correctly claiming your orgasm proudly as your own. Yes, that is exactly what I want you to do.

Why do I make such a suggestion? My reasoning goes back to the fact of the vulnerable male ego, which is especially defenseless when it comes to things sexual. Also, please remember, dear Younger Sister, that a woman's ego strength is such that the placement of credit for her (or her man's) orgasm has no effect on how she feels *as a woman.* You can give away this credit and suffer no damage to your sense of self. You do not want or need to receive "credit" during sex. Rather, you want physical pleasure and emotional closeness. By contrast, your Good Man needs that credit. To be told by you that he deserves full credit for inspiring you and bringing you to your orgasm (of whatever kind) makes him feel incredibly happy, powerful, potent, sexual, successful, and respected.

Hear this now, my sweet American Geisha: *Nothing* makes your Good Man feel better about himself as a man than to know that he inspired and created the orgasm experienced by this wonderful, beautiful, sexual woman, you, his Good Woman. *Nothing.*

Your Good Man could receive a million-dollar bonus or be promoted early or be acclaimed as an outstanding architect. Any of those events would no doubt make him feel great. But when he makes you come on his cock, fingers, or tongue, nothing else (not money, not promotion, not acclaim) makes him feel so great *as a man.* Let me say it again because it is so important to your long-term, loving relationship. When you *enthusiastically* and *consistently* give your Good Man complete credit for your orgasm, he will never leave you, because he feels—you make him feel—so incredibly good as a man.

Another caution. Much as we women may think that men can be insensitive at times, there is one area in which a man is very sensitive: the extent of your enthusiasm for sex with him. A Good Man wants you to be into sex with him. If he senses a lack of real enthusiasm and passion from you, he will be dissatisfied with the sex the two of you have. Let your passion and enthusiasm be sincere and clearly expressed, so that he feels your total involvement in sex with him.

Full-Credit Phrases

Here are some phrases that implicitly or explicitly give your Good Man full credit for your orgasm (spoken either before the orgasm or after):

"Your cock (fingers, tongue) feels so good."

"Fuck me! Harder! Deeper!"

"I love your cock (fingers, tongue) in me."

"I love coming on your cock (fingers, tongue)."

"Oh, god, I love your cock (fingers, tongue)."

"I married you for your cock."

"Nobody's ever fucked me like you do."

"I love how you fuck me. Put it in again."

"How many fingers (in me)?"

"Don't stop. More. Please. I need your cock."

"You make me come so incredibly."

"Put it in. I need your cock." (After he excites you with his fingers and/or tongue.)

"Your cock is (feels) so hard (so big, so thick)."

"Your cock sends (takes) me to heaven."

"Your cock is too big. I can't take any more."

"You always make me come. I love you."

"I come so incredibly with you."

"I need more cock, please!"

"I've never felt like this with anyone else."

"I've never come like I do with you."

"I've never come like this before."

"I've never come so hard (so many times)."

"I want you to fuck me all night."

"I love it when you make me 'shoot.'" (More about female ejaculation in Chapter 5.)

"I've never screamed like that in my life."

"Your cock (fingers, tongue) drives me crazy."

"You fuck me so good (so nicely)."

"The vibrator's not enough. I need your cock (fingers, tongue)."

"Your cock is so good to me."

"Your cock (fingers, tongue) makes my vagina feel so good (excited)."

"My vagina loves your cock (fingers, tongue)."

"My clitoris loves your cock (fingers, tongue)."

"You make me such a sexual animal."

"You're an animal! God, I love it."

"You make me so wet."

"Yes, yes. I'm coming. Baby, oh, baby... I'm coming." (Talk to him as you come.)

"You destroy me (with orgasms)."

As a general rule, be noisy in bed. As I said a few paragraphs ago, let him know that you are really into sex with him, that you are his enthusiastic lover. Tell him how good you feel. Moan. Breathe heavily. Scream. The verbal feedback he gets from you not only lets him know he is pleasing you mightily, but also excites him and gets him harder. And it encourages him to give you even more cock (fingers, tongue), which will drive you even crazier, until you come and make him so happy. Beyond "happy," your feedback makes him so proud of himself, so proud of his cock. You've made him feel fantastic as a man.

With a Vibrator, Where Does the Credit Go?

The Younger Sister in training to be an Asian Geisha is instructed that she *must* follow the directions of her Older Sister Asian Geisha, even when the Younger does not understand *why* the Older is telling her to do certain things as part of her training. I hope you have noticed that I do not take such a strong position as to give you "directions." Rather, I offer "suggestions." And I try to explain why I make certain recommendations. You probably understand and agree with my reasoning for giving away credit for your orgasms to your Good Man, and to do so sincerely and with enthusiasm. Remember that your Good Man always wants to feel appreciated by you, always wants to be your hero, especially regarding your orgasm and total sexual satisfaction and exhaustion.

I wish now to walk a step or two further along the Path to Giving Away Credit for your orgasms. You might, Younger Sister, ask me about a situation involving a vibrator or other sex toy. *What do I do,* you might ask, *if I come wonderfully hard, perhaps even female ejaculate, on my Good Man's cock, fingers, or tongue (or the three in some combination), but added to the mix of what made me come was a fantastic little (or big) vibrator that drove my clitoris into ecstasy and, truth be told, was the proximate cause of my coming so hard and satisfyingly? Help,* you might say, *what should I do about credit in that case?*

This is an important question because I believe that vibrators (and dildos and other sex toys, but *especially* vibrators) should be on your bedside table and always well-charged and available for your lovemaking (not necessarily always used, but frequently). You want your Good Man to be comfortable with vibrators as you incorporate them into your sex life with him. A while ago my husband suggested to me that the old saying about diamonds being a girl's best friend was wrong, that the truth is that *vibrators* are a girl's best friend. I had to agree with him that I'd give up my diamonds long before I'd part with my Pocket Rocket vibrator. You know from masturbating alone with a vibrator how wonderful they are as sex aids to bring you stimulation and orgasm. God, they're fantastic!

What about credit for a vibrator-triggered orgasm? My answer is short, definitive, and covers all situations: "Never give credit to the plastic (or the rubber or the metal)." Instead, of course, *always* give full credit for your orgasm to your Good Man and his cock, fingers, or tongue. Although the vibrator will often (even *most* often, I should think) be there, in use, during lovemaking, it receives zero credit from you for your excitement and orgasm. "Flesh" always gets full credit; "plastic" always get zero credit. You don't want your Good Man to feel that his cock is in competition with your vibrator. Your Good Man is your *lover*; the vibrator is only your (and his) *friend*.

I certainly don't mean that you should lie to your Good Man, and I don't want you to give him credit so as to manipulate him into believing falsely that his flesh caused your orgasm. Instead, I suggest that you always, *as a matter of your sexual policy*, focus on your Good Man's physical organs (his flesh) as the primary causes of your excitement: his cock, his fingers, his tongue/mouth. As useful as the vibrator or other toy can be in increasing your stimulation and intensifying your orgasm, believe sincerely, enthusiastically, and consistently that it is *totally* the flesh of your Good Man's body that has excited you and brought you to orgasm, even to female ejaculation. Is this a fully logical and scientific way of assessing the causes of your orgasm? Of course not. Is sex with your Good Man a fully logical and scientific endeavor? Please answer with me, dear Younger Sister, "Of course not." In fact, sex with your Good Man is a physical and emotional experience. I suggest you respond physically (with a fantastic orgasm) and emotionally (with expressed love and thanks to your Good Man for being the kind of person and lover who makes you come so incredibly).

Men love it when you express appreciation for anything they've done for you. But no appreciation is better received than the sincere appreciation you give to your Good Man for making you come so magnificently.

A Further Step along Your Path to Giving Away Credit

Let's just walk one further step along your Path to Giving Away Credit. When you masturbate alone, with or without a vibrator or other sex toy, also give your Good Man 100 percent credit for the resulting orgasm. How do you do that, since he wasn't even there? Let's imagine a scenario. He has driven off in his truck to a housing development two hundred miles away, where he'll be installing cable and wiring for the next week. You are alone in the apartment you've shared for the last five months, ever since you became engaged, got your .78-carat diamond ring (the exact size of *my* engagement diamond), and set a wedding date. On your second night alone, after talking with him on the phone, your horny animal instincts miss his arms around you, the hair on his chest, his hard cock. So you put on some soft music, take a warm bath (watch that candle!), slip on a sexy silky something, apply baby oil to your clitoris, vulva, and vagina, then masturbate until you come hard with a huge vibrator you and your Good Man call "Mister Big."

When he calls again the next evening, somehow the conversation comes around to the fact that you masturbated the night before. I suggest to you, dear Younger Sister, that the following (or something similar) is what happened last night and is how you tell your Good Man about it: "I miss you so much, baby. I miss your cock in me. I got so horny for your fingers on my G-spot. I thought of us making love all day, your tongue on my clitoris. So I took a nice, warm bath and put on one of your favorite silk teddies and used Mister Big to help me. I imagined your tongue all over me and your cock pounding to the back of my vagina, your arms holding me so tightly, our lips crushed against each other's. And I came so nicely. And then I fell asleep in heaven. Thank you, baby. I love you. Come home soon. You make me feel so good."

Yes, even when he is not there, give him full credit for making you come. His flesh *always* gets full credit. It is your wonderful relationship with this incredible Good Man, his cock, his fingers, and his tongue that make you come *every time* you come. I believe this *is* emotionally true for you, even if the only physical presence was of a vibrator, not of his flesh. I want you to believe this sincerely, enthusiastically, and consistently. As well, your Good Man wants you (and him) to believe this sincerely, enthusiastically, and consistently. When you give full credit to him (and he takes full credit), he will welcome and be happy and relaxed with the idea of incorporating vibrators into your lovemaking and with the idea of your masturbating, both when he is away and, occasionally, when he is lying there right beside you, probably touching you a little, and watching you come with your own version of Mister Big.

Make Him Feel Like a Hero

This chapter has dealt with one way to make your Good Man feel good as a man: by giving him full credit for all of your orgasms. Your Good Man will love you even more for any ways, sexual or nonsexual, that you make him feel good about himself. Essentially, every time you express appreciation for anything he does for you, he feels like a hero, which makes him feel good as a man. Find ways (sincerely) to make him your hero. Even taking out the trash has "hero" potential. You ask him, "Sweetheart, could you take out the trash when you have a chance, please." Later, when you realize he's taken the trash out, say to him, "Thank you, baby. That was so nice of you. I appreciate it." Now he can, and will, think of himself as just a little bit of a hero to his appreciative woman. Your Good Man wants to feel *needed* by you, *important* to you. When you let him know that he *is* needed and *is* important, he feels so good as a man.

To keep your Good Man in love with you and energized in your relationship, do everything in your power to express sincere appreciation frequently to him so that you make him feel wonderful about himself. And the very best way to do that is to give away credit for your orgasm... to him. Make him feel better and better about himself as a man. And he'll be so happy to see his Good Woman becoming more and more of an American Geisha.

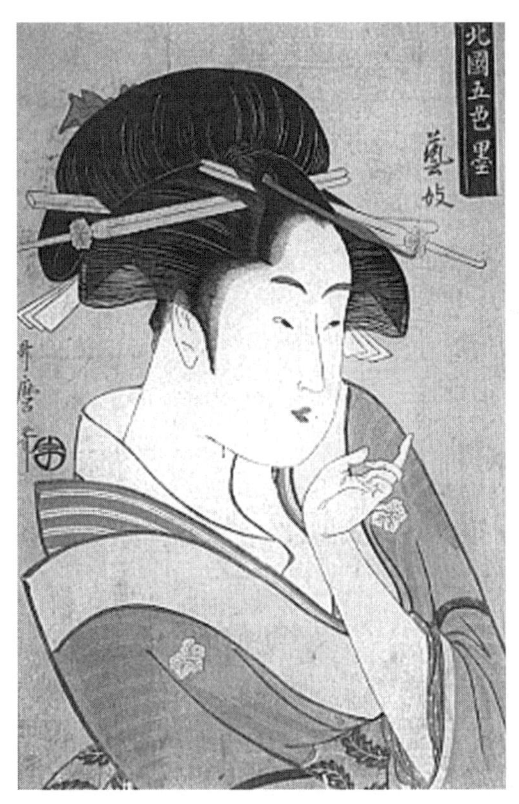

CHAPTER 5

Find Your G-Spot and Learn to Female Ejaculate

With a happy, serene smile on my face and a sleepy, satiated look in my eyes, dear Younger Sister, let me make clear to you, from my own earth-shattering personal experience and from my conclusive research, that the existence of the G-spot and female ejaculation is settled physiological fact, a discovery that can lead to the most intense pleasure and orgasmic release you will ever experience in your life! If that's not worth a heartfelt "Gee!" (as in "gee"-spot) I don't know what is.

In this chapter, you will find and learn to stimulate your G-spot and will become that most feminine and sexual of American Geisha: a female ejaculator, a "shooter."

Let me start by clearing up one commonly held misconception: The ejaculate you forcefully emit is a clear, somewhat sweet liquid that I call Gräfenberg Juice (after the doctor who clinically identified the G-spot). It is definitely *not* urine or even remotely related to urine.

A Most Outrageous Description of My Ejaculation

The G-spot and female ejaculation really do exist. I know. I'm a female ejaculator, a "shooter." If you, dear Younger Sister, are among those who are still unconvinced of this physio-sexual reality, this will be a life-changing chapter for you. Your sex life will never be the same, my oh so fortunate reader. I want to clearly convey to you my experience with female ejaculation, hoping that as I express myself you will both recognize the reality of this phenomenon and begin to imagine the possibilities for yourself. Here I tell my story in an open, explicit way that makes you feel like you are there, almost experiencing my ejaculation yourself.

Sometimes my husband, Rich, and I will be making love without any intention of my ejaculating, and then the idea will strike one of us. We'll start to adjust our lovemaking to go in the direction of having a "shooting" orgasm, as we usually call it. Other times Rich might say, "Tonight is your night, baby. I want you to shoot into my mouth." That excites me. But we never put pressure on me to ejaculate. It's perfectly okay with both of us if I don't. A lot of trust is involved in a G-spot, shooting orgasm, especially when you are doing it the first few times. You have to trust yourself that you can do it (but with no pressure). You have to trust that your partner will not have a negative reaction. At one point you'll have to trust that the familiar feelings of needing to pee are in fact the feelings of imminent female ejaculation, not at all related to peeing.

My pubococcygeus (PC) or vaginal muscles (see Figure 4 on page 95) are well-toned and strong. This is a necessary conditioning to undertake in order to be able to generate the muscle pressure that ultimately provides the force behind the squirting of your feminine juices. For me, it takes a lot of foreplay and specific types of sexual stimulation before I am ready to build toward ejaculation. Although I have often ejaculated on Rich's cock or tongue, I find that having between two and four of his fingers in my vagina provides the easiest way for me to have a shooting orgasm.

Rich might begin by using his mouth and tongue on my inner vulval lips, on my clitoris, and inside my vagina itself. His hands caress my breasts and nipples. After seven to ten minutes, I'll start to use my current favorite vibrator, the Pocket Rocket, on my clitoris, while Rich continues to pleasure me orally. Of course, all of this could lead fairly quickly to a "regular," clitoral orgasm. For the G-spot orgasm, however, this is just the beginning of building my sexual excitement. I may ask Rich to "put it in," or he may decide himself to switch from oral stimulation to inserting his cock in me. Usually he does this from such a position that I can easily keep the vibrator on my clitoris, for example, with me on my back and him somewhat on his left side. Rich may tease me and tell me that I'm too tiny and he can't get his cock into me. He massages my inner vulval lips with his cock, only entering my vagina by half an inch to an inch; then he fully withdraws and again presses his cock against my vulval lips. I go crazy and beg him to fuck me. He teases me like this for three or four minutes. I try to thrust against his cock, to engulf it with my excited vagina. But he pulls back deftly, almost dancing away from my insistent vagina, yet always keeping his hard cock in contact with my vulval lips. I pound his back with my fists and scratch his skin with my nails. But he won't put it in.

Then, right after saying again that I'm too tight to fuck, he suddenly plunges totally and deeply into me, to the back of my vagina. After all the teasing, his cock feels so good. He'll just stay there at the back of my vagina, sort of resting, for twenty or thirty seconds. For me, this is a sexual excitement plateau. After his teasing and then his single thrust into me, I am so excited, and I'm adjusting to having his cock in me. I continue using the vibrator. As Rich starts to move in and out of me with long, deep, slow thrusts of his cock—sometimes switching to what we call "hard and deep" thrusts—I could easily move to a very satisfying vaginal orgasm. (Even as I write this, I am excited enough to masturbate to orgasm rather than to finish writing these paragraphs... but I won't.)

By this time, fifteen to twenty minutes have gone by. We'll come to a point where I say, "Fingers," or where Rich decides to take his cock out, and (with more lubricant) put one or two of his fingers into my now relaxed and open vagina. Using his right hand, he positions it so that the pads of his fingers face my vagina's anterior wall (front wall; if I'm lying on my back it's the upper wall). My G-spot is located here, about an inch and a half inside my vagina. He's able to feel my G-spot easily because my sexual excitement has caused it to swell and become quite palpable to the touch. He will probably track the rough top of the G-spot area, then slide one finger down the left side of the G-spot and the other down the right side. A good amount of pressure from his fingers awakens my G-spot's sensitivity even more as he holds it between his two fingers and slowly, deeply rubs it.

Rich may insert a third and even a fourth finger into me, continuing to rub *with pressure* over the G-spot area. My excitement rises. My PC muscles are sensitive and flex some, particularly at the back of my vagina. Rich will pull all four fingers totally out of my vagina, then thrust them strongly back in, then again apply pressure (especially with the longest, middle finger) to my G-spot. By now we've been making love for twenty-five to thirty minutes, and I am getting hotter and hotter from so much stimulation, especially of my G-spot. The deepest of my PC muscles, at the back of my vagina, are twitching and flexing, eventually beyond my control, so that as my orgasm occurs the muscles constrict at the back of my vagina, where Rich now tries to thrust his fingers. The PC muscles close so tightly around his fingers that they shut off the deepest part of my vagina and force his fingers toward my vaginal entrance. Rich resists this pressure and pushes back with his fingers, which only excites me to a desperate level of needing to push even harder as I now both reflexively and consciously squeeze my

PC muscles. The sensation is like I'm trying to close nearly the full length of my vagina and expel his fingers. Eventually he can no longer resist the muscular closing down of my inner vagina, and his fingers come flying out. The incredible pressure of my PC muscles also squeezes a reservoir of Gräfenberg Juice that lies in a spongelike organ near my vulval lips. As his fingers exit my vagina, they are immediately followed by the Gräfenberg Juice, which seems to explode out of me with the same force that expelled Rich's fingers.

This warm liquid (which is definitely *not* pee) covers Rich's right hand and lower arm, and my entire vaginal area, thighs, and ass. Rich quickly flips his body around and puts his mouth totally over my vagina, his tongue probing deeply, to cause a second gush to flow into his mouth, where he either holds it to show me or swallows it so that his tongue can probe again for more of my love juices. At times, I experience multiple orgasms and multiple ejaculations, all within moments of each other, expelling almost enough ejaculate to fill an eight-ounce coffee cup! (Some women claim to be able to release as much as a cup and a half.) Especially after multiple shootings, I am exhausted both physically and emotionally and cannot move, totally destroyed by the intensity of my orgasms. My brain doesn't work. I sleep. "Please, Rich, respect my orgasm," I say. That means, "Leave me alone, please." I'm in heaven.

The Most Intimate Sexual Experience of His—and Your—Lives

Let me promise you that as an American Geisha you will be able to offer to your Good Man the most intimate sexual experience of his life as you give him full credit for inspiring you to come on his cock (or fingers or tongue) with such animal force and intensity that a stream of nearly clear, pleasant-tasting ejaculation fluid floods into his eager mouth or covers his cock, balls, and thighs. If left unhindered, your love juice can even shoot several inches or *several feet* into the air, before showering back down onto the bed and soaking the sheets in the most feminine rain imaginable. (One of my girlfriends reports that her ejaculate has reached her ten-foot ceiling, more than six feet above her bed.)

The Asian sex secret I reveal to you here is that, incredible as it may sound, the fact of female ejaculation is well-documented in Japan from at least the sixteenth century. It is reflected in art forms of that period, including drawings and woodcuts that portray ecstatic women at the explosive moment of release of their warm, liquid love lava, and also depict containers for catching the fluid (see Figure 1 for an example).

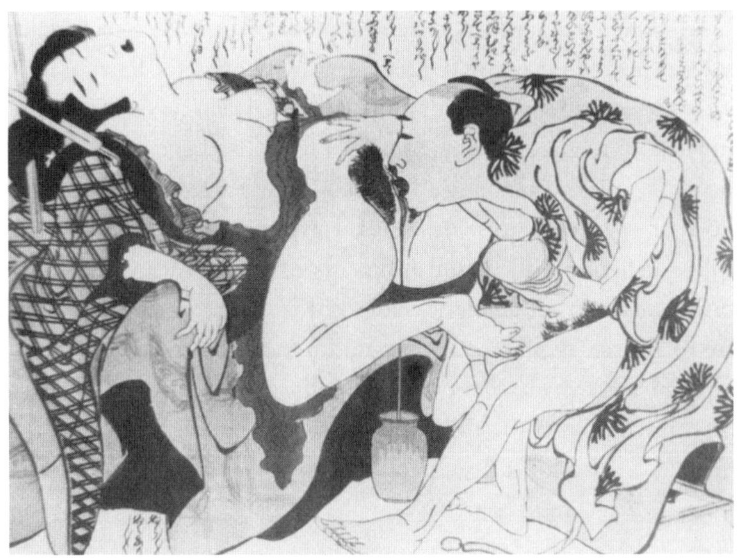

Figure 1. A Japanese woodcut depicting a man holding a container to catch female ejaculate. *Reprinted from* Erotique du Japon.

How could so many of us in the West remain ignorant of the G-spot and female ejaculation if they have been well known for so long ago in the East? The truth is that in the West, female ejaculation *was* understood as a physiological fact as far back as pre-Christian-era Greece and Rome, as recorded in writings. And much earlier than that, India and China recorded descriptions of women's feminine waters.

Was it the Dark Ages of Europe that erased the West's memory of this dimension of a woman's sexuality? Was it Western religion's difficulty in coming to terms with the full sexual capacity of women? Or was it something else? Whatever the reason for this memory lapse, your Older Sister American Geisha wishes to convey to you that female ejaculation is not a shocking, extraordinary finding of the late twentieth century. The Eastern world has practiced this technique for many hundreds of years. It is time to make it widely known again in the West, time to allow Western women their birthright to fully experience their natural capacity for a fulfilling sex life that includes G-spot orgasm and female ejaculation.

These facts of female physiology and sexuality somehow stayed lost to Western medical awareness until the early 1980s, when several independent investigative groups reported that there did exist an acutely sensitive area along the anterior (front) wall of the vagina. It came to be known as the G-spot, named in 1982 after the German physician Ernst Gräfenberg, whose generally ignored 1950 paper described the spot, behind which resided another organ of exquisite sexual pleasure, the female prostate (see below).

So mysterious are these sexual hotspots that even today many Westerners doubt their very existence. Or they believe that female ejaculation is somehow only possible for the equally mysterious Asian woman. Such nonsense. Every woman has a G-spot (of varying size), and 90 percent can ejaculate. (About 10 percent seem to have a G-spot that is too small to accommodate the stimulation necessary to bring about "the gush.") The solving of the mystery of the G-spot may surprise you even more than the mystery itself, my Younger Sister. I'll explain as simply as possible.

A Reservoir of Love Juice

To understand what the G-spot represents, we must take a quick, imaginary trip back to the womb. Imagine that the uterus holds two fertilized eggs: twins, a boy and a girl. In the earliest stages of development there is little to visually differentiate the developing boy and girl. In fact, at one point both embryos will seem to have female sex organs; it is not until later in development that the introduction of the hormone testosterone will cause the boy to develop a penis and testes, much as estrogen will much later enlarge the preteen girl's breasts during puberty. The male embryo eventually develops a prostate, which at full maturity (reached during puberty) will secrete a seminal fluid that, when mixed with sperm from the testes, will flow into the man's urinary tract and be ejaculated out of his hard cock upon orgasm.

Likewise, the female embryo, of course, develops the sexual organs of a woman. The organ that in the male embryo becomes the prostate develops in the woman into what has been called the Skene's glands, after Alexander Skene, M.D. In 1880, Skene described the glands and their ridged ducts as urological structures surrounding the female urethra, and as having little if any function; most often they were only noticed, he wrote, when they became infected and created a urological problem. However, by the 1950s it was recognized that this tissue had erectile qualities: It hardened to the touch. It is the Skene's glands, particularly the series of parallel ridges on the glands, that can be felt *through* the front wall of the vagina, especially as the glands' erectile tissue engorges with blood and hardens during stimulation of the G-spot from *within* the vagina. The Skene's glands (the G-spot

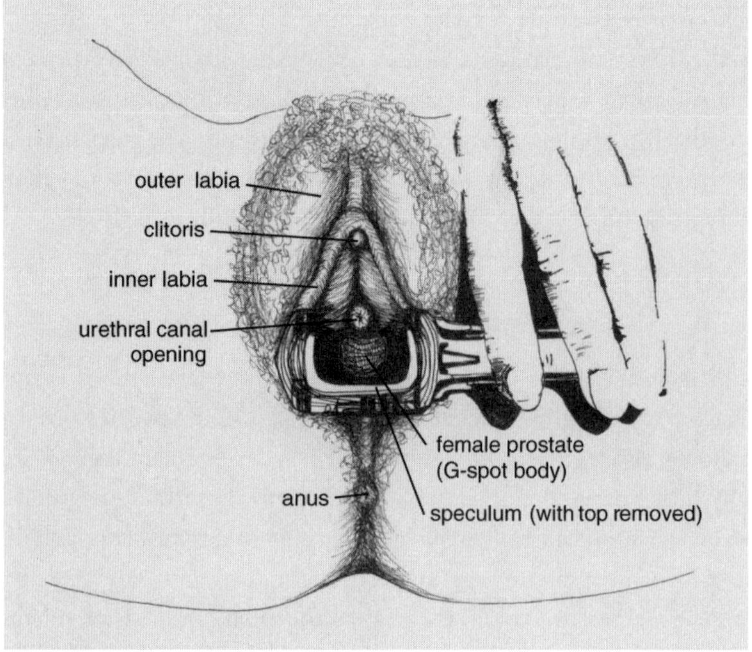

Figure 2: Front view of the G-spot. *Artist: Moti Melchizedek. Reprinted from* Female Ejaculation and the G-Spot, *by Deborah Sundahl.*

body) have now been more properly renamed in the medical community as the female prostate (see Figure 2); they were recognized in the 1980s as an organ of sexual pleasure, *not* simply as a urological structure.

As an American Geisha who will soon be familiar with your own female prostate, you will have an understanding of this incredible element of your femininity and sexuality that few Western women possess. (All women possess the organ; few women possess the understanding.)

Are you surprised? Your Older Sister American Geisha certainly was when she first understood with clarity the existence of the female prostate gland. It is a fully accepted medical fact that the female embryo develops a gland similar to the prostate that develops in the male embryo. As you directly stimulate the G-spot with cock, fingers, tongue, or even a specially shaped vibrator or dildo, the stimulation passes through the wall of the vagina to the female prostate, causing it to engorge with blood, to grow

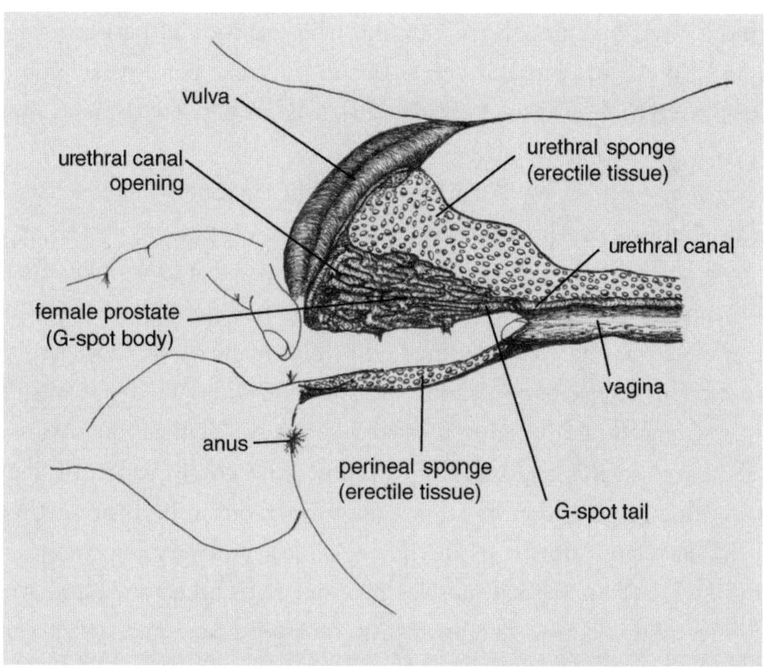

Figure 3: Side view of the G-spot. *Artist: Moti Melchizedek. Reprinted from* Female Ejaculation and the G-Spot, *by Deborah Sundahl.*

larger and harder, until it is readily felt from within the vagina. In addition, a liquid with properties somewhat similar to the male seminal fluid begins to accumulate in a reservoir called the urethral sponge, a four-inch-long area of spongy tissue surrounding the urethra and the female prostate (see Figure 3 on the previous page).

Women and men started life as identical embryos, and as sexually mature adults, both can have an orgasm that involves ejaculation. The male seminal fluid is transferred by ducts from the prostate and is ejaculated through the urinary tract and out the tip of the cock. The woman emits from the female prostate a similar fluid (but in much larger quantities than the man), which also leaves the body through the urethra. Powerful muscle contractions occur around the urethra, causing the ducts of the female prostate to open into the urethral canal. (Imagine the Grand Coulee Dam in Washington State, another type of reservoir, opening its gates and pumping copious amounts of water into the Columbia River under incredible pressure.) The woman's warm love juice (Gräfenberg Juice) exits under enormous pressure through the urethra, which is located between the clitoris and the vaginal canal. It comes out in the same place where you pee, but rest assured, dear Younger Sister, that it is *not* pee, but rather a mostly clear, pleasant-tasting nectar.

You may wonder, my American Geisha in training, why you have not had this shooting or squirting experience before. Or perhaps you think you may have had such an experience, but you dismissed it as a fluke. Or perhaps you mistakenly thought you had peed and had no interest in pursuing such an embarrassing event any further. I think many of you have never experienced female ejaculation simply because you didn't realize it was there to be experienced, didn't realize it existed, didn't realize that you possess the sexual organs to make ejaculation possible (the combination of female prostate, ducts to the urethra, and spongy reservoir around the urethra to hold the ejaculate prior to its discharge). A last and very important, even critical, factor: Your vaginal muscles may not have been toned and strong enough to create the muscle tension and intense pressure necessary to expel the ejaculate so forcefully as to be unmistakably noticed by both you and your Good Man partner.

The PC Muscle Group: Your Love Muscles

The Asian Geisha knows that to please her man she must spend many hours in training, learning various forms of entertainment, as well as always seeking to increase her sexy femininity and beauty. The American Geisha knows, too, that she must work hard to be as sexy, feminine, and beautiful as possible, including keeping her body in a toned, fit condition. It is particularly important for your and your Good Man's utmost sexual pleasure to work to tone the most feminine of muscles, those that are involved in the G-spot orgasm: the vaginal muscles known as the pubococcygeus (pue-bo-cox-uh-gee-us) muscles, which are located in the pelvic area. These PC muscles—which I call the vaginal muscles or love muscles—surround and support the area of a woman's body from her clitoris in the front to her anus at the rear. Among several other muscles in that area (including the anal sphincter muscle), it is specifically the PC muscle group that is engaged when you bear down to stop the flow of urine. This most common use of the PC muscle group will make it easier for you to identify and isolate the muscles when you seek to exercise them, as you must do in order to female ejaculate.

Much of your success in experiencing both incredible orgasmic release and powerful ejaculations is related to the strength of the PC muscles when they're relaxed. The American Geisha wants to have strong, toned love muscles. Happily, nature has made it very easy to strengthen the PC muscles simply by exercising them—and there's no need to coordinate your workout clothes with your cross-training shoes before you go to the gym. You can exercise your PC muscles while seated at your desk, while in the car, even while chatting with some hot potential Good Man or while walking your dog. It's that easy. Anywhere. Anytime. In private. In public. And no one will know. Pretty sexy, huh?

In the early 1940s, Arnold Kegel, M.D., an Ob/Gyn practicing in the Los Angeles area, designed a simple PC-muscle-toning exercise for new mothers who were suffering from urinary incontinence. Practicing what became known as Kegel exercises not only helped women to strengthen their urinary control, but also, serendipitously, led many to report greater sexual satisfaction for themselves and their husbands. Perhaps someday Dr. Kegel and his exercises will be remembered and acknowledged more for his contributions to sexual health and happiness than for urological health. You, sweet Younger Sister, now know that the two, the sexual and the urological, are not so different and separate as one might think when it comes to the mysteries of the G-spot, female ejaculation, and incredibly satisfying sex.

Three Hundred Times a Day

Dr. Kegel's PC muscle exercise is easy to perform. Simply squeeze and hold those pee-controlling muscles for five to ten seconds, then relax them. Repeat this in sets of twenty-five, fifty, seventy-five, or one hundred, according to the time available to you, until you have completed three hundred contractions of your PC muscles. Do this each day. Within two weeks you will almost certainly notice a difference in the tone of the muscles and in your response to sex. Happily, your Good Man may also notice a marked increase in your vagina's tightness around his cock. Ah, heaven to a man: A tight vagina that closes firmly around his cock and provides greater friction to excite him to orgasm! Your man will also love your ability to squeeze those muscles at will while he's inside you, providing his cock with a very stimulating pulsing sensation.

These love muscles will bring such sexual joy both to you, Younger Sister, and to your man. Squeezed just slightly, tentatively, they tease your man's cock; held more tightly, they seem to encase his cock and to tighten and shrink the size of your vagina, making his cock feel larger to both of you. Finally, after many minutes and much buildup of sexual tension, and with your PC muscles passionately contracted to their fullest extent, they will cause your vagina to seemingly try to turn itself inside out as they tighten around your man's cock (or fingers or tongue). These exquisite contractions seem to drive his cock toward the opening of your vaginal canal. As he pushes back (and push hard he must or those mighty love muscles will expel him from your vagina quickly and forcefully), your muscles, now beyond your willful control, continue to push against his insistent cock. The two of you reach an ecstatic but unsustainable and precarious balance.

The moment of your ejaculation is only a desperate twenty to sixty seconds away. He applies renewed pressure to your G-spot in order to drive your love muscles into the final involuntary contraction that will shoot his cock (fingers, tongue) out of your vagina. This is followed by a bursting forth of ejaculate from your urethral canal opening, which occurs under the pressure of both the "uncorking" action of his cock and the spasming of your toned and strong, well-exercised love muscles. Again and again the PC muscles squeeze the urethral sponge reservoir until all the Gräfenberg Juice has been expelled and absolutely soaks the bedsheets. Wow! You are one hot, sexy, ejaculating American Geisha lady!

Men Love Your Ejaculation!

Both my personal experience and my research show that your Good Man love partner (or future Good Man love partner, if you haven't found him yet) will be both surprised *and* pleased by your ability to gush forth large amounts of feminine fluid. However, it is probably best to prepare him for the experience rather than to surprise him with an eruption of your feminine fountain in the midst of your normal lovemaking. Let him know that you have been learning about female ejaculation and have been practicing alone, and have had some success, and now want to share the experience with him. Earlier I suggested that you buy a fresh, unmarked, unhighlighted copy of this book for your Good Man. Now I suggest that you point out the relevant chapters and ask him to read about the G-spot, the female prostate, and female ejaculation.

You want to educate your Good Man so that he is aware of and comfortable with these facts. The two of you might share your joint wonder at the revelation of this new information and its potential to add to and deepen your sexual ecstasy and intimacy. You will also want to tell (and show) him how to stimulate you to an ejaculatory orgasm. He'll appreciate knowing how to perform well rather than being left alone to try to figure out, for example, how best to find and to stimulate your G-spot. He'll be an eager learner. Of course, when the two of you have successfully brought you to a shooting orgasm, you will give him full credit for motivating and stimulating you to incredible heights of sexual and emotional satisfaction.

Thank him. He'll feel so good as a man that his cock (fingers, tongue) produced such an incredible, spectacular orgasm for his woman. If your Good Man is like mine, he'll happily volunteer to sleep on the large, now-cold puddle of ejaculate juice so that you don't accidentally roll over onto it. That makes him a double hero. Thank him again.

How to Female Ejaculate

You've read enough, dear Younger Sister, about the results of female ejaculation. Now it is time to discover your G-spot and its related sexual pleasures. Get naked on your bed, comfortably prop up your head and shoulders, and put a pillow under your butt. Use lubricant as necessary, but not too much. To locate the G-spot, insert the middle and index fingers of one hand just a very short distance (one to one and a half inches) into the vagina, with the pads of the two fingers flat against the front wall of the vagina (the side toward your belly button). It can be difficult to distinguish the G-spot area from the surrounding tissue when you are not sexually excited; it can feel very much like the rest of the anterior vaginal wall. As your finger pads (particularly that of the middle finger) press *firmly* again the front wall of the vagina, moving slowly, you may begin to become excited, with the area of the G-spot becoming fuller. You may notice a spongy area against your two fingers. Push firmly against this spongy area while *slowly and rhythmically* moving your two fingers repetitively in a "come-here" motion, as though you were calling someone to you. The G-spot area will become more defined and obvious as the female prostate (on the other side of the anterior vaginal wall) becomes engorged with blood. Its "ribs" or ridges become more pronounced in response to your massage of the G-spot.

As you continue this stimulating massage, the G-spot area will protrude into the vaginal cavity. How much it protrudes varies in different women from subtle to substantial, probably due to varying sizes of female prostates and varying erectile responses to the massage stimulation. Use the gentle pressure of your two fingers to explore, through the vaginal wall, the dimensions of your female prostate. Feel the ridges on top; slide your fingers down the left and right sides, sort of holding the organ gently between the two fingers. Notice the responses to your fingers' pressure in different areas

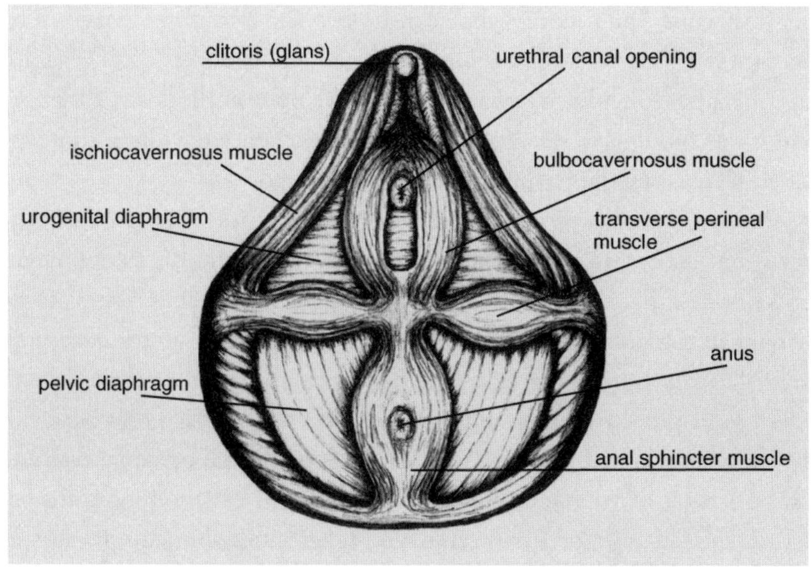

Figure 4: Muscles of the pelvic area . *Artist: Moti Melchizedek. Reprinted from* Female Ejaculation and the G-Spot, *by Deborah Sundahl.*

along the top of your female prostate; the sensations can vary from erotic to neutral to even slightly painful. Over time and with increased sensitization, all the areas will yield erotic feelings.

Where Is the PC Muscle Group, Exactly?

Because the PC muscle group is so important to the G-spot orgasm and ejaculation, we need to learn a little more about it—a little more knowledge that will lead to incredibly more sexual and emotional pleasure. First, let me define the PC muscle group in a way that may help you to envision it in your body. Let's again look at its full name: pubococcygeus muscle group. As the name implies, it is not a single muscle, but rather a group of muscles that work together, in unison (see Figure 4). They are involved not only in orgasm and ejaculation, but also in initial arousal and vaginal lubrication. (Men have PC muscles too, and they serve essentially the same functions in them, except for the part about vaginal lubrication, of course. In men they're also involved in creating and maintaining erections.)

The word "pubococcygeus" can be broken into three parts: pubo-coccy-geus. "Pubo" (from the Latin) means "pubic and." "Coccy" (Latin, but originally from Greek) refers to the coccyx bone at the base of the spine (which was thought to resemble a cuckoo's beak, hence the Greek root word *kokkyx*). "Geus" (more Latin) means "pertaining to."

Putting these three definitions together, we find that the pubococcygeus muscle group is "a group of muscles pertaining to the pubic and coccyx bones." Said another way, this muscle group stretches from your pubic bone in the front all the way to your tailbone (coccyx) in the back, a distance of perhaps five to seven inches. It traverses in a figure eight from the area of your pubic bone, mound of Venus, and clitoris back past both sides of your urinary opening, past both sides of your vaginal opening, even back past both sides of your anus, finally attaching to the coccyx bone at the base of your spine. It supports the rectum and other internal organs. It measures in thickness anywhere from one-half inch to over two inches.

Because this muscle group is so long, it is served by two major nerves. The front two-thirds (toward the clitoris) is associated with the pudendal nerve, which responds to stimulation around the clitoris, labia, and vaginal entrance. The back one-third of the muscle group (toward the coccyx) is associated with the pelvic nerve, which connects to the bladder, uterus, urethra, prostate (male and female), and lower spinal cord. Strictly clitoral orgasms (which involve only the pudendal nerve) are not accompanied by female ejaculation. When *both* the pudendal nerve and the pelvic nerve are excited, however, orgasm can often include female ejaculation.

Clitoral and G-Spot Orgasms Are Different

Are you sensing where this little anatomy lesson is going? Younger Sister, one of these nerves (the pudendal) sends messages of sexual arousal from the clitoris to the brain, resulting in a *clitoral orgasm,* which involves contraction of the front two-thirds of the PC muscles. The other nerve (the pelvic) senses the G-spot stimulation of your female prostate and seems to send those messages of sexual excitement, at least in part, to a different, more primitive (may I say more animal and probably more emotional?) part of the brain, the brain stem, resulting in what has been called the *G-spot orgasm* (or *female prostate orgasm* or *blended orgasm*). With practice, female ejaculation can quite frequently accompany the G-spot orgasm ("blended" because it incorporates neural messages sent through both the pudendal and pelvic nerves). You'll want to reread this section a few times to put a picture clearly in your mind.

Yes, my dear American Geisha in training, you are capable of two different types of orgasm, orgasms that not only follow different neural paths to (probably) different parts of your brain, but also are qualitatively different. That is, you experience the two types of orgasm, the clitoral and the G-spot, differently. They are *not* the same. For much of the twentieth century Sigmund Freud had many women believing that their clitoral orgasms were "immature," and that the mature woman could experience a vaginal orgasm (though Professor Freud never did diagram or otherwise explain how the woman could actually experience that "mature" vaginal orgasm). The 1960s brought the feminists and the love children, who said Freud was wrong and that all orgasms are fundamentally clitoral orgasms, which are not "immature" at all.

Now we know that, indeed, there are two *different* orgasms, the clitoral orgasm through the pudendal nerve and the G-spot orgasm through both the pudendal and the pelvic nerves. Though I would hesitate to declare Freud "right," there is much anecdotal evidence that the G-spot orgasm is often more satisfying to a woman than the clitoral orgasm, involving as it does both a deeper and a more emotional experience. I can only suggest that you, my Younger Sister, experience many of both types and ascertain for yourself the relative orgasmic merits of each.

I Leave You with a Tease

There seems to be a third and extremely powerful type of orgasm, though rarely experienced by the great majority of women: the *uterine orgasm*. It is effected through the pelvic nerve (alone, unblended) and depends upon deep, strong thrusting of cock or finger (or super-long tongue) that "jostles" the cervix and indirectly stimulates the uterine muscles (a part of the

PC muscle group). The resulting orgasm, experienced more fully in the brain stem, seems to have the most intense emotional component, and is usually so totally satisfying that you'll be completely satiated by just one. This orgasm is much less likely to involve female ejaculation. I reference this orgasm again in Recommended Readings, at the back of the book.

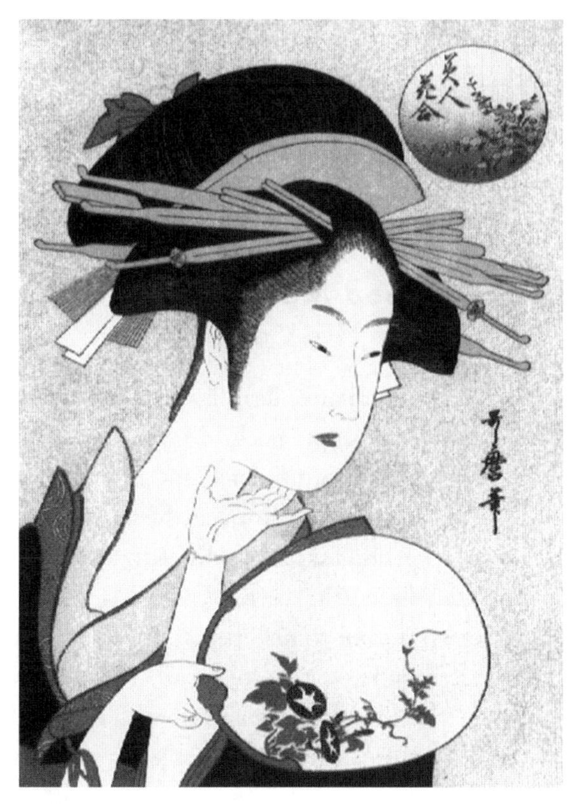

CHAPTER 6

Worship His Manhood

The Asian Geisha is always very concerned with the image she conveys, for a positive image brings her more business from better clients. As an American Geisha your image in your Good Man's eyes is of considerable importance to you, too, my Younger Sister, for a positive image brings you greater love and commitment from him, and more quickly. For this reason I ask that initially in your relationship with your Good Man you avoid most of the slang or profane terms for lovemaking, breasts, and vagina.

Let Your Good Man Know You Love His Cock

There is, however, one key alternative term I want you to become comfortable with early in your relationship: "cock." I believe that your Good Man has an association between the word "penis" and the act of urination that makes the term "penis" not nearly so erotic as the term "cock." Remember this: A man pees with his penis and makes love with his cock. From the beginning in any intimate relationship with a Good Man, refer boldly, sweet Younger Sister, to his "cock," not to his "penis." If he should inquire about your use of the term, let him know that for you there is an erotic, sexy association with his "cock" that you don't experience with the word "penis." Tell him that when you look at his naked body you see his cock, not his "penis." Ask if he understands and agrees with you. I think he will. Let him know, however, that you prefer the terms "vagina" and "making love" to the alternatives, because the slang words are so often used in the context of anger and swearing rather than in the context of intimate lovemaking. You are too much a lady, *at least in the initial stage* of your sexual relationship, to be comfortable with low-class references to such a beautiful act as lovemaking, yet too sexual and passionate to think of your Good Man's cock as simply a urological instrument. (Later in a sexual relationship, you might want to begin to use "cunt" and "fuck" as alternative expressions, according to your joint preferences.)

The Asian Geisha knows that, essentially, a man and his cock are really one, that much of a man's psychological identity—his ego—is bound up in his cock. When you, as an American Geisha, massage his cock you massage his ego; when you love his cock, you love him as a man. Nothing makes him happier; nothing ties him closer to his American Geisha than the fact that you always build him up, in his own eyes, as a great, worthy, potent man.

Fairly quickly after your relationship with your Good Man becomes sexual (and remember, you *only* become sexual with someone who is a "Good Man" for you; see Chapter 10), you should express to him that you love his cock. In fact, an American Geisha will often express love of her man's cock *before* she is ready to express love of the man himself. If you are married or in a committed monogamous relationship, you express love for both the man and his cock. Say with sincerity such things as:

- "I love how your cock feels."
- "I love how your cock makes me feel."
- "I love what your cock does for (to) me."
- "I love your cock in me."
- "I love how your cock makes me come (or 'shoot')."
- "I love coming on your cock."
- "I love how hard your cock is in me."
- "I love just to look at (touch) your cock."
- "I love your cock, hard or soft."
- And, simply, "I love your cock."

(*Caution:* Be sure you do not convey that you love cock *generally*. Rather, make clear that *his* is the cock, the only cock, that inspires you to the point of expressing such love.)

Create a Shrine to His Cock

After many expressions of your love for his cock, create a shrine of some sort to convey to him that you "worship" his cock. The Asian Geisha engages in many rituals, some in the presence of her men (the tea ceremony being a familiar one) and some while she is away from them (such as the rituals involved in preparing her face and clothes). These rituals convey to her clients the great respect she holds them in, for instance as she pours a client's tea with focus and exaggerated ceremony. The American Geisha, dear Younger Sister, engages in similar, if somewhat different, rituals regarding her face and clothes. The rituals of creating a shrine and of worshipping his cock (not in any religious sense, of course) are a ritualistic expression to your Good Man of how powerfully you are affected by his sexuality and how much you respect and love his cock.

Your own creativity is probably your best guide as to what the shrine to his cock will look like. Although the Asian Geisha may have a small religious altar or shrine near the entrance to her home, I suggest that you build your American Geisha shrine to your Good Man's cock in your bedroom. Here are some elements you might consider including:

- A naked photo of him, framed
- A close-up photo of his cock (hard or soft)
- A collage of photos
- A photo of you sucking or holding his cock
- A drawing of his hard cock
- Incense
- Candles
- A recirculating water sculpture
- Small rocks
- A short poem or note to his cock
- A single fresh rose or other flower
- A small plant
- Perhaps simply a framed sexy photo or collage of photos (including you, naked) hung on the wall

The idea behind your shrine is to let your Good Man know how much his sexuality inspires you (and, of course, that you've never been so inspired by any other man). Occasionally light a short stick of incense at the shrine, or otherwise show that you "visit" the shrine, so he will know that you actively use it when you acknowledge or meditate for a moment or two on his cock and on your relationship with him. Replace the poem or note in the shrine every now and then, and tell him to read the new one when he has a chance.

You Love His Cock Like No One Ever Has

Here's the true test of your love for your Good Man's cock. At some point after you have responded so excitedly and orgasmically to his cock, after you have so often expressed how much you love and want his cock, after you have created a shrine to his cock, he will say to you these *exact* words (I promise, with no doubt at all in my mind): "No one has ever loved my cock as much as you do." It will be true, too; no one ever has. In fact, no one ever *could* love his cock like his American Geisha. And if he is the right Good Man for you, you love *him*, too; you love the person he is. Nothing could be better for him. You love his cock and you love him. To your Good Man, this means that you love him totally, both his sexual self and his unique personality. Wow! On top of all that, you are beautiful; and you squirt; and you are nice. He'll never leave you. Where would he go? There is *no one* like his outrageous, incredible, beautiful, and feminine American Geisha!

I really *do* worship my husband's cock and I really do tell him so, often. My "shrine" to my husband's cock is in the form of a mounted and framed photo collage that includes naked XXX-rated photos of us (each alone, and together) and little notes from me, as well as fun, sexy, R-rated photos of him. It hangs on a wall just four feet from our bed. When certain people visit (including all children) I take it down; when others visit, I leave it up. I'm proud of worshipping my husband's cock. And, yes, he has told me many times, "No one has ever loved my cock as much as you do." And I know he is right, that no other woman could ever love his hot, sexy cock so well as his American Geisha wife.

More Ways to Show Him How Much You Love His Cock

After your Good Man's orgasm, he is as exhausted as you are after your shooting orgasm. The French call the orgasm *le petit mort,* "the little death." Understand if he has no more energy to pursue sex, cuddling, or small talk with you. Know that you have killed him (temporarily), that you have given him a most beautiful, satisfying little death. Let him sleep the sleep of the dead. Let him enjoy what you and your vagina (mouth, hand) have given him. As he showed respect for your orgasm, so should you for his. Perhaps slip out of bed and return with a warm, wet washcloth to lovingly, worshipfully wash his cock and balls and belly. Careful! His cock is so sensitive to touch after his orgasm.

Your vagina is already shaved, naked, and beautiful. No doubt he loves the White Tigress hairless beauty of your uniquely exquisite sexual organs. After a short while of being sexual with this Good Man, tell him that because you love his cock and what his cock does for you, you want to be able see his shaved and naked cock and to feel his smooth, naked skin against your smooth, naked skin. Tell him you want to lick and suck his naked balls. Add, too, that when he pounds his cock so deeply into your naked vagina for such a long time, which you love for him to do, you sometimes become somewhat raw and irritated by the cutting action of the hair of his cock against your naked, tender vaginal skin. Emphasize honestly that you love to be able to see and touch his cock, hard or soft, unencumbered by a forest of hair. Tell him you want him to keep the masculine pubic hair above his cock (trimmed, perhaps), and shave only the cock and balls. Tell him it makes you feel sexy and wet just to imagine his naked cock against your naked vagina. Later, ask him to shave his cock and balls *daily* as part of his routine facial shave or while he showers, so that the sharp, stubby, day-old growth on his cock does not irritate your vagina. Here's another truth that will motivate him to shave: Once the hair on the cock and around the base of the cock is removed, his cock looks bigger, longer, even more sexually stimulating to you.

Ask yourself, "Could my Good Man ever love me *too much?*" Go ahead, ask yourself this question, right now, as you are reading. What is your answer? I believe you answered, "No, of course not." Could your Good Man ever tell you too often, "I love you"? Again, of course not. You want to be loved and to hear it, to know it from him, often. (Am I right?) Well, your Good Man is the same way about this as you are, but regarding his cock. Know this, my Younger Sister American Geisha: Every man wants to know that his Good Woman loves his cock; you cannot tell him this too often (as long as it is sincere each time). When you tell him this he feels good about himself as a man, feels happy, feels connected to and loved by you. He will love *you*, in part, because you love his *cock*. If you do love what his cock does for you, scream with ecstasy when you come on his cock (or fingers or tongue), but also *tell* him with words that you love his cock (or fingers or tongue), and tell him often. (Excuse me a moment, I've got to go find my husband and tell him I love his cock, his fingers, *and* his tongue.)

Focus on his cock as the Asian Geisha focuses with exaggerated intensity on her tea ceremony or on refilling her client's empty sake cup. Hold his cock, hard or soft, in your hand. Examine it from just inches away, transfixed by its power over you. Stroke it slowly, feeling its skin under your gentle fingers. Kiss it lightly, all over. Lick the frenulum (the sensitive underside of the cock just below the head) with the wet tip of your tongue. React when your attention makes his cock twitch, begin to harden, or become rock hard. Your Good Man loves it when you enthusiastically pay close attention to his cock. He even loves it when you just *look* at his cock.

The Asian Geisha knows how simple men are, how happy they are when a beautiful, bright, cultured geisha devotes herself totally (again, most of the time, nonsexually) to making her clients feel so interesting, so witty, so smart—in short, the center of her attention. The American Geisha realizes, too, that her Good Man's ego is a simple thing that doesn't need much to make it happy and content. Sex is a factor for the American Geisha, of course, but, as we discussed in earlier chapters, any way that you can make your Good Man feel good about himself *as a man* will bond him to you. Be sincere. Be supportive. Build him up. And don't forget to love his cock. Do all of this and he's yours forever.

Your Good Man Always Risks Rejection

The Asian Geisha tries always to be gracious and accommodating to her clients. If they request her presence at a meeting, party, or convention, she will try very hard to do what she can to attend the function, perhaps shortening her time at an earlier event or adjusting the time she plans to arrive at a later function. She does not want to disappoint her clients by being unable to accommodate them. The roles of client and geisha are such that if the client makes a request of a geisha with whom he has had a long-term relationship, he has some expectation that she will accede to his wishes; that is, he presumes to a certain extent that she will do as he requests. For the geisha's part, she, too, likely has the same understanding: that it is her duty to make every attempt to accommodate her most important clients.

For the Asian Geisha it is just good business. Were she unable to make adjustments to her schedule in order to please an important client, he might well feel rejected. And this could damage their relationship. The client may want to avoid the risk of rejection in the future by visiting a different teahouse and pursuing a relationship with another, more accommodating geisha.

From the earliest days of dating your Good Man through years of marriage to him, it is inherent in his being a man that he constantly risks rejection by you. Early in the relationship you may turn down a date, not want to go to the restaurant or movie he suggests, refuse his good-night kiss (even on the third date, as I foolishly did to the man I later married), not let him come into your home, not want to have sex. We've already talked about how fragile a man's ego is, and yet your Good Man has the courage to keep taking the initiative with you, proposing things to you that you might turn down, thereby rejecting *him* in the process of rejecting his idea or suggestion.

Respect your Good Man's courage in the lifelong journey of risk-taking that he embarks on with you. It takes balls to be a man. Real nerve. Respect that. Even after you are together, even married, his risk-taking continues. A man's life always involves a risk of rejection. It's bad enough that he faces that risk at work (as do you, too, of course), but he also faces it at home, even from you, his Good Woman who loves and respects him.

At work, a man may risk rejection (of an idea, a project, a request, a report, an opinion) that could negatively impact how he feels about himself as a man. However, a man's greatest psychological vulnerability is not the risk of rejection at work, but the risk of rejection at home, from you, his Good Woman. A man's ego is most vulnerable when, after you have established a sexual relationship, he tells you that he wants to make love to you. At that point you hold his ego in your hands.

If you refuse his invitation or request for sex, you may think that you refused for some objective reason, such as the late hour, illness, chores that need doing, your own distractedness, not enough time, hunger, the baby's diaper, not in the mood, or a hundred other reasonable scenarios that preclude lovemaking at that moment. If he were to ask why, you'd say, "Nothing personal; it's just ____________ (fill in the blank)." You probably wouldn't see it as a big deal. "We'll make love later," you'd probably think, if you thought about it any more at all.

For him, when you refused his (brave, risky) offer to make love, you refused his cock. Translation: You refused him as a man. He feels bad about himself as a man, refused by his girlfriend, fiancée, or wife, rejected by the woman he loves, his cock rejected by the woman he loves, his manhood refused and rejected.

"Wait a minute," you might think, "I'm tired/it's late/we have to leave in twenty minutes. That's why I said no. I'm not rejecting him or his cock. I love him and I love his cock."

What Is an American Geisha to Do?

I'll put it simply. An American Geisha *never* refuses or rejects her boyfriend's, fiancé's, or husband's cock, just as an Asian Geisha tries never to refuse her client's requests. Rather than a refusal or rejection of his cock, always try to be enthusiastically ready and available to your boyfriend, fiancé, or husband whenever he wants to make love with you. It is good, dear Younger Sister, that he wants you, that he is attracted to you, and that he wants to put his cock in you, even if for some reason his desire is a bit inconvenient in its timing. Always make it a priority to have the time and energy to be your Good Man's enthusiastic lover.

So, your *first thought* upon being asked by your Good Man to make love should be, with full enthusiasm, "Yes." Go for it. Truly be enthusiastic. In fact, a Good Man only wants to make love with you when you are truly enthusiastic. Again, try to have a sincere enthusiasm when he wants to make love with you. He, his ego, and his cock can all sense when you are not enthusiastic. And they take it badly and personally when you are not really into making love with the three of them. Show real enthusiasm whenever you make love with your Good Man.

If there is some reasonable factor that mitigates against a ninety-minute love fest, your *second thought* should be to suggest some other sexual activity:

- "Great. Can we make it just a quickie? I'm a little tired."
- "Okay. I'm a bit tired. You just go ahead. Put it in."
- "Sounds good. I'll leave for work in fifteen minutes."
- "Great. Let me just suck you, right now."
- "Good idea. Just a little bit now. We'll finish up later, okay?"

Your *third thought* may be the one you most often actually use. In this situation you cannot make love enthusiastically or even hurriedly. You just plain cannot make love now, perhaps because of a time problem, an illness problem, even a transient mood problem. Or a just-got-home-from-work-and-can't-switch-gears-that-fast problem. It really doesn't matter what the problem is; if it is there and the first two approaches don't work for you, then it cannot be gotten around and you will not be making love right now.

Still, Never Say "No"; Instead, Make a Date

But your Older Sister said *never* to refuse or reject your boyfriend's, fiance's, or husband's cock. Yes I did. And you will not refuse or reject that Good Man's cock that wants to be inside you. Remember, if you refused or rejected that enthusiastic cock, your Good Man would tend not to see the situation reasonably ("Oh, she can't make love because she's feeling achy all over. Okay"). Rather, he'll tend to think, "She doesn't want my cock, she doesn't want me in her, she doesn't love my cock or me, she doesn't like how I make love, and she doesn't even want me." Holy cow! All you said was you were a bit ill. Nothing more. Well, I told you earlier about the vulnerable male ego and its particular sensitivity when it comes to all things sexual. If I have exaggerated some or quite a bit here (and I *think* I have, but I'm not sure), that silly Good Man of yours is still hurt at least somewhat by your refusal and rejection. Deal with it. He's a guy. He doesn't take that kind of thing well. So, your job, dear American Geisha, is to help your Good Man as best you can to know that you haven't refused or rejected him. You've simply been unable through Thought Number One or Thought Number Two to find a way to make love to him right now.

Say, "I'd love to make love with you now, but I'm achy all over." This tells your Good Man that you are attracted to him and *do* want to make love, but *can't*. Once he knows you'd "love to make love," he can be more receptive to your reasons for not doing so *at the moment* ("I am achy"). So far so good, but not enough, dear Younger Sister. Next, propose a date to him, for instance, "I should be all right in an hour or so. I'd like for you to be inside me then. Is that okay?" Or, "I know I'll feel better in the morning. Can we set the alarm a half hour early and make love then, honey?" Even better, when you can, add a little something special to the date you propose, such as, "I'm so exhausted tonight. Can we go to bed early tomorrow night and make love then? I'll wear my new garter belt for you, baby."

Try to see your refusal/rejection of sex with him from his perspective. Men are so simple. He's like a little boy whose mommy won't buy him a toy. "You don't love me," the little boy pouts as he catastrophizes and generalizes ("You don't love me") from a simple, specific event (mommy not buying a toy). Younger Sister, when it comes to dealing with the "toy" that hangs south of your Good Man's belly button, you should know that he is still a child, still catastrophizing and generalizing and pouting ("She doesn't want my cock") over the specific event of your being too achy to have sex at the moment. You've heard it before: Men are such little boys. Yes, they are, especially insecure and vulnerable about their cocks. A feminist might jump up on a soapbox and lecture your Good Man about his immaturity and insensitivity to your honest concerns about being achy. I confess that might be a fair approach to take, but, I propose, it is not as loving, understanding, and *powerful* as the approach I'm suggesting.

Do what I'm suggesting and you'll have a happy, smiling man looking forward to the date that you've proposed. Since you only postponed and didn't refuse or reject sex with him, he does not feel rejected or unwanted. In this more positive frame of mind, he can take his focus off of himself and his hurt feelings and may even ask, "Can I do anything to help you with the aches, sweetheart? Maybe I could massage your legs. Let me see if we've got some rubbing alcohol." Again, if I exaggerate a bit, can you at least agree with my point, Younger Sister?

You become more and more of an American Geisha when, instead of refusing and rejecting your man, you take the following steps in a positive, loving manner:

1. Say, "I'd love to make love with you, but (give your reason)."
2. Propose a date (not too far in future).
3. Add something special (sometimes).
4. Ask, "Is that okay?"

A last word on this subject. Let me emphasize that I am not asking you to *manipulate* your Good Man with this approach. What I've proposed is an honest, caring way of handling a situation in which, for one reason or another, you cannot make love at the moment. Please explain this entire approach to your Good Man; even have him read this chapter. And seek his agreement that it is a loving and caring and sexy way to handle those times when you cannot make love. An American Geisha is proud of how she conducts herself in her relationship with her Good Man, and she hides nothing from him. Your Good Man will love you even more because he appreciates your confident assertiveness and total refusal to manipulate him.

The more you love and worship your Good Man's cock, the more and more you are becoming an American Geisha.

Part Three

Planning for Marriage

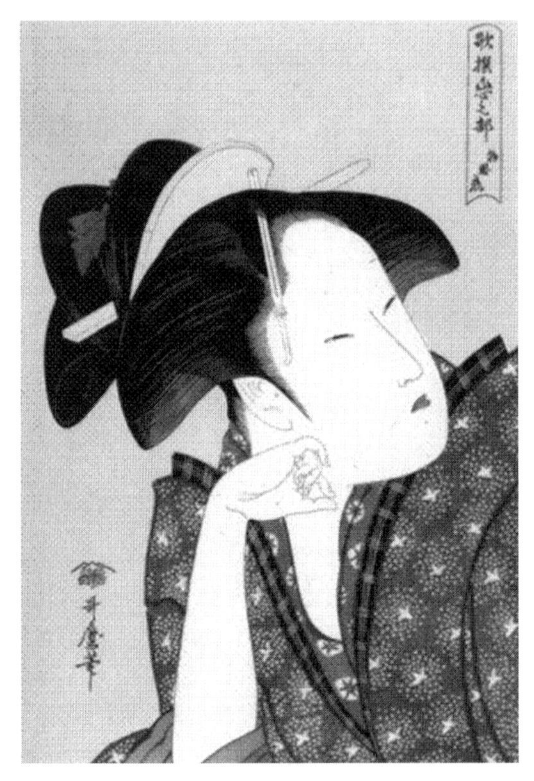

CHAPTER 7

Define Your "Good Man"

A confident, hot, sexy woman, whether an Asian Geisha or an American Geisha, knows that she needs and deserves only a Good Man in her life. She has much to offer to the right man and thus can be choosy and require that he have admirable qualities to bring to the relationship. The Asian Geisha holds out until she finds the right man to be her *danna,* or patron; the American Geisha holds out for the right Good Man to be her husband. The stereotype about Asian women that says they can be very focused and determined to get what they want is another positive stereotype that all women need to take advantage of, especially in the realm of love and marriage. Do not give in and accept less than you deserve. Hold out for what you reasonably need from a man, your Good Man.

Once you have re-created yourself as a confident, sexy, beautiful, and feminine woman, you will attract men to you. And then you'll have to choose the ones you want to favor with your company. Right now, you need to define for yourself what a Good Man is so that you'll know which ones to date and which one to marry.

This chapter will help you to define the basic characteristics of a "Good Man," encourage you to start becoming aware of what you want in a relationship, and educate you about the importance of spending time only with Good Men.

My Story

I had a tendency to leave things up to fate. Like many Asian people, some part of me accepted that my destiny was foretold in the zodiac and that I just had to passively wait for events to unfold in my life. I did a terrible job of finding men. If I'd had a love and marriage plan, I never would have wasted so much time with men who were not Good Men for me. Though I knew I wanted marriage and children, the two longer-term relationships I had (with Scott for three years and Neil for five years) were with men who didn't want to marry me or to have children, and who both ultimately got involved with other women before we broke up.

Scott and Neil might have been fine for someone who didn't want marriage, babies, love, or much sex, but neither was a Good Man for me and my needs—reasonable needs, I think. The truth is that during my eight years with Scott and Neil I was not very aware of what I really wanted in a relationship with a man.

I was involved with men who didn't appreciate my kind personality and who didn't tell me I was pretty. I asked Neil what kind of woman he wanted to date, hoping to hear, "You're my type." Instead, he replied without hesitation, "I'd like to date a thin woman." So often Neil's insensitive words hurt. Again, I was foolish, desperately staying with men who treated me badly.

After Neil left for Korea, my mind remained unclear about him for two more years. While he was living in Korea, I held out hope that he was looking forward to marrying me when he came back. That was a total illusion. He was dating a Korean woman while I was waiting for him in Los Angeles. I thought that he would be faithful to me even though he never mentioned any future plans with me or made any promises. Only my total lack of consciousness and clarity about the situation allowed me to hold on to the illusion that Neil loved me and would someday return to marry me. I was such a mindless fool. I wasn't clear about my fundamental needs. All I knew was that I wanted to be married and have a baby. Foolishly, I didn't think beyond that. I wasted years of unhappiness and loneliness because I never really focused on whether or not the men I was with were good for me.

Time Is of the Essence

Although there are many different traits you might look for in a man (and you'll consider lots of them in the next chapter as you put together your love and marriage plan), I want to first suggest four specific areas in which I believe a man must live up to a high standard in order to even be considered by you as a possible Good Man for you to date and marry.

As an American Geisha, you are seeking long-term happiness in a good marriage, so you do not want to waste any time dating or being in a relationship with a man who is not a Good Man for you, and who therefore has no chance of winning you and becoming your husband. The familiar saying "Time is of the essence," which can be traced back to the *I Ching* book of wisdom, means that time is important and shouldn't be wasted. This is true in your search for your Good Man. You should not waste your precious time with men who are not Good Men for you and with whom you'll never enter into a marriage relationship. You need to determine as quickly as possible whether or not someone is a potential Good Man for you, and from there decide whether or not to pursue the relationship.

The biggest time-waster for you on the road to love and marriage, as it was for me, will be the time you spend with inappropriate men. I spent years and years with the Wrong Men. Please learn from me, bright Younger Sister. Do not spend *any* time with a man once you realize he is not a Good Man for you.

The Four Core Characteristics of a Good Man

As you consider what makes a Good Man good, you will first be concerned with the very basics. These are the most important and fundamental areas of a man's character that must be right in order for you to have a wonderful, happy love relationship and marriage with him. The smart, assertive, sexy American Geisha does not compromise at all in these four areas; your Good Man must show you that he possesses these traits.

A Good Man's Four Core Characteristics are:

1. He has good values.
2. He is aware, conscious, and responsible.
3. He is nice, and he is supportive of you.
4. He is positive, optimistic, and happy.

1. A GOOD MAN HAS GOOD VALUES

What this means, in essence, is that he is honest, that he tells the truth to you and to others, in both his personal and business lives. Because he tells the truth you can trust him and relax in the security of the relationship. You do not always have to be on edge, wondering what the truth of any situation actually is. When people live in accordance with their values, they have integrity.

A man can have good values no matter which religion he practices (or even if he practices no religion). Liberals and conservatives, Democrats and Republicans, rich and poor can all have good values. When a man tells the truth you can respect him. The American Geisha would find it difficult to respect a man who lied to her, and respect for your husband is critically important in a good, happy, sexy marriage. Both Scott and Neil were less than fully honest with me, and I realize now that I didn't always respect them.

2. HE IS AWARE, CONSCIOUS, AND RESPONSIBLE

Your Good Man is conscious of what is going on around him, of his relationship with you, of his dealings at work, and, generally, of the passing of the years and events in his life. When he is aware and conscious you feel heard by him, appreciated by him for what you do and who you are, connected to him because you are both actively involved in your relationship. For your Good Man to be responsible simply means that he doesn't blame others for much that happens in his life, but instead takes it upon himself to do the best he can to succeed in life and in his relationship with you. He's dependable.

Here, again, I now see that both Scott and Neil, rather than taking responsibility for doing what needed to be done, chose to deny that they had serious untreated problems (erectile dysfunction and depression, respectively).

3. YOUR GOOD MAN IS NICE, AND HE'S SUPPORTIVE OF YOU

Niceness or kindness is so important in the definition of a Good Man. Couldn't you, dear Younger Sister, put up with a whole bunch of imperfections in a man if he were consistently the nicest person in the world in the way he treated you? "Nice" is an underappreciated adjective when it comes to personality traits. Notice whether he treats other people kindly, too.

A man who is supportive of you has your best interests at heart and wants you to be successful in whatever you attempt. He believes in you, cares for you, and wants you to be happy. He builds you up and never tears you down. He's a friend and a teammate as well as a lover and a husband. I see so clearly now that Scott and Neil just weren't very nice to me.

4. HE IS POSITIVE, OPTIMISTIC, AND HAPPY

This final core trait has to do with a Good Man's way of looking at the present and the future, as well as how he interprets the events of his past. Many psychologists believe that this attitude has a strong genetic or inherited element that is difficult to change. Most basically, you want to be a happy woman who's sharing her life and marriage with another happy person, not a happy woman trying to make her unhappy husband happy. Getting someone else to change is always difficult, even harder if much of his negativity is based in his DNA.

From my experience with Neil, I can testify to the intractability of depression and negativity, no matter what another person does to help the sufferer overcome it. Instead of your changing him for the better, his negative life view will probably drag you down—at least, that's what happened to me. Over the years with Neil, I became more negative, more pessimistic, more depressed, and unhappy. I blamed myself that I couldn't help him no matter what I did.

As a kind, caring person, dear Younger Sister, encourage such a man to find help—as difficult as any change may be—but do not try to be a helpmate to him and do not put your own happiness at risk by staying with him. Instead, find a Good Man who has done the psychological work he needed to do. Find a Good Man who is already positive, optimistic, and happy.

The Asian Geisha accepts all of the men she deals with exactly as they are, without demanding, expecting, or even hoping that they will change. She knows that they will not. Learn this lesson, my dear American Geisha: Men will not often change. Do not try to change a Bad Man or a Wrong Man, for only your great unhappiness is likely to result. I felt lonelier when I was with a Wrong Man than I did when I was actually alone. Don't make my mistake. Instead, find a Good Man who *already* has the core qualities that you require for your and his great happiness together.

What If You Choose a Bad or Wrong Man?

Your American Geisha Older Sister likes to stay positive in her advice to you, dear Younger Sister. However, to make the point of how important a

Good Man's Four Core Characteristics are, I need for just a moment to get a little negative. Imagine that instead of seeking a Good Man who embodied these four important personality traits, you became involved with a Bad Man or Wrong Man who embodied their opposites.

Your life with this man might entail serial lies, some big, some small, perhaps about where he was, whom he saw, what he did. Perhaps even criminal behavior. You'd worry, be unsure, insecure, anxious, upset, perhaps angry or scared. Since he's also unaware, this Bad Man doesn't know the real you, who you are at your core. Perhaps debts mount and he's not conscious of your family's precarious financial situation. His lack of consciousness and responsibility does not make him a good employee or otherwise enhance his job security; nor does it bode well for his being a dad, if he has even given serious thought (awareness) to parenthood. And blaming others (the government, his boss, *you*) rarely is a good strategy for having a happy, successful life or marriage. Perhaps this Bad Man will be unsupportive of you, put you down, and treat you unkindly, because he is not a nice person, not a nice man, not a nice boyfriend, not a nice husband. You'll feel insecure, perhaps even physically afraid. Finally, if Mr. Bad Man is negative, pessimistic, and unhappy or even depressed, imagine what that does for your day-to-day quality of life together!

Remember this, please, Younger Sister: If a man lives his life from bad values, if he is irresponsible, unkind, or very negative (any *one* of these four problem areas), you want no type of relationship at all with him. You do not share your heart, your vagina, your bed, or your life with a Bad Man. If you can avoid it, don't even share a cup of coffee with a Bad Man! If somehow you have gotten entangled with this Bad Man, end any such relationship now. If somehow your Mr. Bad exhibits all four of the Bad Man characteristics, you should also spend considerable time analyzing (perhaps with professional assistance) your original choice to date him so you'll never do it again.

Again, if you are with a Bad Man, get out, figure out why it happened, and start looking for a Good Man, only a Good Man. It's not worth wasting your precious time; it's not worth putting your energy into a Bad Man. Because you're worthy. You are a worthy person. You are a Good Woman. You deserve and will find a Good Man. (See the Recommended Reading list for some books that may be helpful if you've wasted time with Bad Men or even just Wrong Men.)

Notice What He *Does*, Not What He *Says*

When you find a Good Man with the Four Core Characteristics—one who is honest, aware, nice, and happy—then your pleasant assignment is to further determine whether other elements indicate that he could become a longer-term dating partner, a sexual partner, and finally a marriage partner.

No man is perfect. The American Geisha knows this and does not seek an impossible perfection in her man; however, she does seek to be with, to date, to have sex with, and to marry only a man who possesses the core characteristics that will support a long and happy marriage to her, a woman who has all of the characteristics of a Good Woman. Your Geisha Consciousness knows that you are so smart and so hot and so sexy that you do not have to consider selling yourself short in terms of the man you choose to date and to marry. He will be a fine man, a Good Man—or else you will not date, have sex with, or (heaven forbid!) marry him.

You will be able to get some hint of whether a man is a Good Man early in your relationship, often without ever going on a date. Look positively and optimistically at any man to see whether or not he has the four core qualities. Keep your awareness and focus on looking for his strengths in these areas, not on actively seeking out his weaknesses (unless his actions indicate that there is something negative to be on the lookout for). Watch for behaviors (that is, not so much what he *says* but what he *does*) that give you indications of how his personality matches up to your four core requirements for your future husband.

Remind yourself that a Good Man has the integrity to act in ways that reflect his professed values. That is, if he has good values (what he *believes*), then his behaviors (what he *does*) are a natural and consistent consequence of those values. Watch out for (and run from) the man who says all the right things, which would seem to indicate good values, but who does not seem to behave or live from those values. A man without integrity between his beliefs and his behaviors is not a Good Man. At least one indication that you are dealing with a Bad Man is the frequency of his apologies for misbehaving, followed soon by more bad deeds and more smooth-talking apologies. Don't *listen* to the apologies; *watch* for the repeated bad behaviors. To treat you this way is abusive. Leave in a hurry; full politeness and gentle partings are not required for such a manipulative, unprincipled Bad Man. A good book on how to recognize and avoid inappropriate men is Sandra L. Brown's book *How to Spot a Dangerous Man Before You Get Involved* (see Recommended Reading).

Once You Choose a Good Man

Once you choose a Good Man with whom to have a relationship, please forever focus positively and optimistically on his good points and strengths, and accept his relatively minor bad points and weaknesses. You want to always be totally supportive of your Good Man, never subtly undermining him with your concerns for his limitations. The smart, sexy American Geisha can only be so accepting if she knows that, at heart, this is a Good Man for her, despite whatever less important shortcomings he may have.

The secret that I impart to you here is that the Asian Geisha, once she and her *danna* have chosen one another, makes his happiness (sexual and otherwise) and her support of him her highest priority, though her actual decision to take on a *danna* is more of a business/lifestyle choice than a love choice. The American Geisha, for reasons of love and support, chooses her Good Man with a clear understanding of who he is, and she does all she can to build him up as a man (sexually and otherwise) both in her eyes and in his own eyes. She then reaps the many wonderful rewards that such a happy and empowered Good Man will bring to her, to their relationship, and, ultimately, to their marriage.

My husband is most definitely a Good Man, but he is certainly not a Perfect Man (remember, there's no such thing). As to the Four Core Characteristics, he has a high sense of integrity; he loves sharing what he calls a "conscious relationship" with me; he is tremendously nice and supportive; and he's the most consistently positive and optimistic person I've ever known. He has his faults, though. He reads the newspaper two hours a day, without exception; he has a very relaxed attitude toward work and money; he is more of a thinker than a doer; and he wants, at age sixty-three, even more sex than I do. I accept and even support that he is this way, and it doesn't detract from our love relationship, because at his core my husband is a Good Man. Dear Younger Sister American Geisha, when you find a Good Man, please accept and support in him those aspects of his personality that you may not prefer, but which are not critical to defining him as a Good Man. He'll love you for both your acceptance and your sincere support.

Remember, though, at the outset of the relationship you must be *very careful* to ascertain that this man truly is a Good Man; otherwise your efforts may ultimately be wasted on a man you cannot marry because he has very different values or is not sufficiently conscious or doesn't treat you nicely or is an unhappy person.

Don't Sweat the Smaller Stuff

Please listen to your American Geisha Older Sister's story of her search for a Good Man as a cautionary tale. I had just finished my five-year relationship with Neil and was determined not to make so many mistakes as I began anew my quest for a Good Man (although at that time I had not yet conceived of the specific qualities that made a Good Man, nor had I even figured out exactly what I needed from a man). I did know that I didn't want a long-distance relationship, and I knew that I wanted someone to marry, an intimate life partner. I wanted someone to have dinner with, to see a movie with, to have sex with; I wanted someone to be nice to me.

I wrote down the following list of what I wanted from the next man I got involved with:

I need a man who...

- makes me feel bigger than I am (I'm small)
- tells me that I am pretty
- is in my future plans
- appreciates me, even my small gestures
- wants me more than I want him
- has a hot body temperature in cold weather
- sees my new red nail polish and says, "That's sexy"
- makes me laugh

- understands my good intentions
- sees my fat body as having a basically good underlying shape
- helps me to wake up at five in the morning to exercise
- supports my different fad diets without any criticism
- is supportive of my writing
- helps my digestion when we're dining together
- sees me as a nice woman
- will be my child's father

As I look at my list eight years later, I am glad that I didn't miss out on the relationship with my husband just because he didn't have a hot body temperature or a sexy response to my nail polish. Nor is he too enthusiastic about 5:00 A.M. workouts or sitting quietly as I jump from one diet to another. I'm not sure if he even understands how he could help my digestion at dinner. I'm glad that when I met my husband I didn't sweat the small stuff.

Now I realize that I should not have defined the Good Man I sought with these less important personality traits. I should have stuck to the basic elements that make a Good Man good, as I'm asking you to do. From there I should have been ready to accept a man (as I did ultimately) who had traits that differed from those of my Perfect Man. I eventually figured out that these differences are not terribly important to a happy marriage. So, please, dear Younger Sister, don't sweat the smaller stuff when it comes to selecting an otherwise Good Man for you.

At the same time, however, as an American Geisha you almost certainly have basic requirements of a relationship, what I call Your Four Fundamental Needs. I will discuss them in the next chapter. Although it is important not to sweat the smaller stuff when it comes to the personality traits of a potential Good Man, it is equally important to be clear about and focused on getting your basic relationship needs met. Just as you want to avoid spending time with a Wrong Man or Bad Man, you also want to avoid wasting time with a man, even a Good Man, who doesn't have essentially the same relationship goals as you do. We'll talk about all of this in more detail in the next chapter, dear Younger Sister, when we develop your love and marriage plan.

You Get to Do the Choosing

Let's talk a little more about choosing your Good Man. So far, I have spoken more about attracting men to you, not so much about your choosing a Good Man to whom you are attracted. It may seem that attracting a man places you in a passive role, because he is the one who chooses whether or not to approach the healthy, slim, and beautiful you. The attitude of the smart, hot, sexy Asian Geisha—and this should be your attitude, too—is that *she* has the final choice to make. She is so beautiful, sexy, feminine, and classy that many men will be attracted to her and she will have the option of choosing among them. You, too, dear American Geisha, should have the confidence that your beauty, femininity, and presence will allow you to choose from among those attracted to you. You can choose one or more Good Men to date who seem to be just right (but probably not perfect) for you, and ultimately you can make the final choice about your one Good Man to marry.

By being a feminine-ist—by operating out of your receptive, feminine self—you happily allow a Good Man to engage in the masculine behaviors of searching and hunting. Though superficially the man seems in control because he is taking the action of approaching you, truly it is you who, knowing the powerful secret of receptive femininity, control the ultimate outcome of the man's behavior.

In Chapter 3, I said that when you increase your options, you are making progress. Think about it. If your femininity and beauty attract men to you in large numbers, this increases your options as you try to assess whether this or that man might be your Good Man. The more options you have in terms of potential Good Men who approach you, the more opportunities you have to find and choose the right Good Man for you. You are definitely making progress toward soon being happily married if you have twenty-six Good Men to choose from rather than only three or one. Increasing your options certainly is progress toward your ultimate goal of marriage to the right man, your Good Man. (Finding your husband is a "numbers game," and if you define for yourself what a Good Man is, the game you play will involve a number of Good Men, not Wrong Men who waste your precious time.)

You Are a Good Woman

We have worked in this chapter to define a Good Man. But we now need to take a moment to look in our mirrors, at ourselves. If we want and expect to attract and to marry Good Men, then we need to be Good Women. Otherwise the Good Man we wish to marry will marry someone else who is a Good Woman.

To know what makes a Good Woman takes no further information than we have already covered. The same Four Core Characteristics of a Good Man are the Four Core Characteristics of a Good Woman. We can simplify the Four Core Characteristics by reducing each to a single word.

A Good Woman is…

1. honest … 2. aware … 3. nice … 4. happy

In order to attract a Good Man who has these Four Core Characteristics, you must be a Good Woman who also exhibits these Four Core Characteristics. Measure yourself against this list, and move toward being more and more honest, aware, nice, and happy.

A Good Man may fuck many beautiful women but marry none of them. The beautiful woman he does marry will also be a nice woman. Be that nice woman. Of course, "nice" for you as a Good Woman and for him as a Good Man does not mean that either of you is unassertive about your own needs and wants in the relationship. It means that each of you has a caring, compassionate way of interacting with one another and the rest of the world.

I want you to use your refrigerator to help you stay conscious and aware of what a Good Man is for you. High up on the fridge, please post the Four Core Characteristics of a Good Man. Photocopy the list from these pages or handwrite your own version. Later I'll ask you to post additional items on your fridge, so clear some space for me, will you please? As your fridge fills up and you become more aware of what you want in your Good Man, you are becoming more and more of an American Geisha.

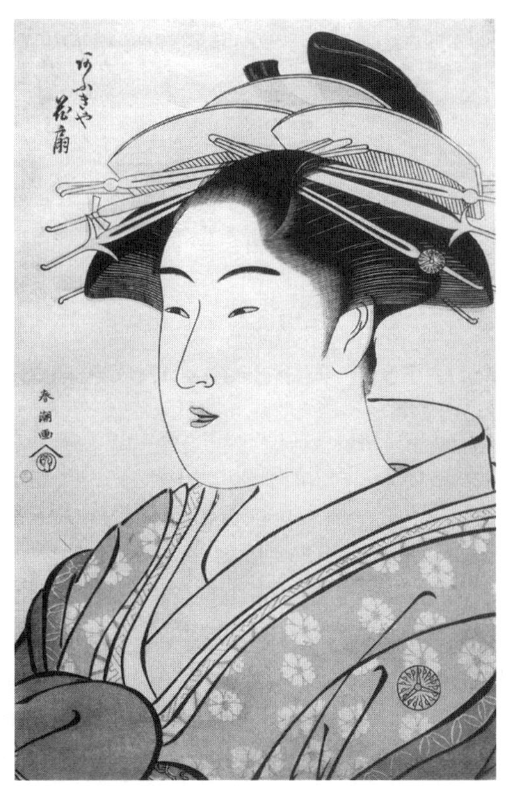

CHAPTER 8

Create Your American Geisha Love and Marriage Plan

I said in the Introduction that this book would be a practical guide that would help you to be married to your Good Man within twelve to eighteen months. I promised that I would suggest specific actions you could take to get you closer to that goal. Now, in this chapter, I need for you to become actively involved in the process so that I may keep my promise. It is time to develop your American Geisha Love and Marriage Plan. Actually expending the effort to create a plan is the most proactive step you can take; then you must put your plan in writing to give it a reality it lacks if it remains only in your head.

Your Four Fundamental Needs

Your Older Sister wants you to start your planning by defining your most important, basic needs in a relationship. You must be clear about these needs, both for yourself and so you can communicate them to men who are possible candidates for your future Good Man husband.

Think about what your most fundamental needs are, write them down, and stay aware and conscious of them. Although your basic needs are certainly for you alone to determine, I believe I can help. If you bought this book, I believe I know enough about you to guess what your essential relationship needs are. See if I'm right. Here are Your Four Fundamental Needs:

1. You need to be married (if true) and to have kids (you decide).
2. You need a strong love relationship (of course).
3. You need a passionate sexual relationship (of course).
4. You need a Good Man, and no other kind, to date and marry (absolutely).

I suggest to you that these four needs are reasonable, achievable, and essential to a happy life with your chosen man. (And a wonderful Good Woman like you deserves a happy life!) You may have other *important* desires (such as where to live, family income goals, compatible religion, travel, time for friends and family, time alone). However, the needs that I call Your Four Fundamental Needs are the *absolutes* that you require from a relationship. And you must internalize them and communicate them, over time, to any Good Man whom you are considering dating or marrying. If any man, even a Good Man, chooses not to accommodate Your Four Fundamental Needs, you should not begin to date him or you should stop dating him, whether or not you have had sex with him. And, of course, you should not marry him.

Remember, not all Good Men want to marry or have children. Not all need a strong love connection, nor a sexy relationship. Just because a man you are dating is a Good Man, that is not necessarily enough. He must also be willing and enthusiastic about meeting Your Four Fundamental Needs.

There will be some of you dear Younger Sisters who do *not* desire marriage or children, perhaps being fully happy with a committed, monogamous, live-in relationship that even in the long term will not involve either marriage or children. Some couples choose to have a commitment ceremony in lieu of a conventional wedding. Some couples will be made up of two women, rather than a man and a woman. Any such arrangement that pleases the two of you is totally supported by your Older Sister. You will simply adapt my suggestions to your particular situation. For instance, the first of Your Four Fundamental Needs may read like this:

1. You need to be in a permanent, committed, monogamous relationship, without children.

Furthermore, as you grow older and reach different life stages, Your Four Fundamental Needs may change, perhaps from the need for a committed relationship at age twenty-three to the need for marriage (and children?) at age thirty-one. These are *Your* Four Fundamental Needs. Adapt my suggestions to the desires and goals that you have at any particular point in your life.

I now realize how important mutual love is to me in a relationship. Over a total of eight years, neither Scott nor Neil (I am so embarrassed to admit) ever said he wanted a future with me. Never. (Neil the brave, at the L.A. airport on his way to Korea, turned to me after he'd walked into the area reserved for ticketed passengers, and, for the first time in three years, said, "I love you." How could I have been so foolish—desperate—as to stay for so long with a man who didn't love me?)

What Do You *Need* and *Want* in Life?

Right now, think ahead to when, within eighteen months (or perhaps just twelve), you are at the altar, marrying your Good Man. Visualize your future, the future of a hot, sexy Good Woman who knows exactly where she wants to be and what she wants. The secret I reveal to you here is that the Asian Geisha knows what she needs and wants out of life. An important part of Geisha Consciousness is that the geisha is aware of her needs and wants in a relationship. Whereas the Asian Geisha specifically *does not* want love and marriage (they would harm her business life), the American Geisha specifically *does* want love and marriage (they make her personal life so happy). The Asian Geisha would discourage men who wished to take the relationship unacceptably far, and the American Geisha would discourage even Good Men who did not want to at least consider the possibility of taking the relationship to love, commitment, marriage (perhaps), and children (possibly).

Think again about the list of things that I believe you require for a happy lifetime together with your Good Man. They are very important, yet so simple. First, assuming this is true for you, you want to be married, not just living together or dating, but married and with children. Second, you will *only* be happy in a strong, healthy love relationship, not in a marriage of convenience or "friendship," but one of true, mutual, emotional love. Third, in proudly honoring your physical, animal desire for sexual as well as emotional love, you want and need a relationship that has a strong sexual, chemical attraction. Lastly, and perhaps of greatest importance, you wish to have this lifetime commitment *only* with a man who is good for you, your Good Man for life.

Read the last paragraph again, please. Don't these four requirements represent what you really *want* and *need* most out of a relationship? Aren't they all reasonable to expect of the man you marry? And, with some effort from you, aren't they all achievable? I hope you can answer all of my questions with an optimistic, confident "Yes!"

An important Asian Geisha secret that all women should know, understand, and use is that the Asian Geisha is a strong, independent woman who knows what she wants and who can be very focused and determined to do what is necessary to achieve her goals. Don't let the stereotype fool you;

Asian women are not as passive and docile as many Americans may think. It is true that Asian Geisha are generally nonconfrontational with everyone, including their male clients. They don't like arguing, fighting, shouting, screaming, or other types of negative, nasty personal interactions. Asian women generally are polite and well-mannered, but do not mistake this for passivity. An Asian Geisha is capable of pursuing what she wants with a quiet persistence and determination, an assertiveness that speaks up, softly, for what she needs in order to be happy.

Likewise, the American Geisha will reasonably discuss and negotiate many elements of her relationship with her Good Man, but she should refuse to compromise on her basic principles or requirements, which I believe are represented by Your Four Fundamental Needs. If a man does not want to or cannot fulfill these needs, he is not the right Good Man *for you,* though he may be a good and fine person, and perhaps a good match for another woman who at a particular time, for instance, may not want love, marriage, or a baby as part of her relationship.

If you have any concerns about whether you can stand up for what you reasonably need and want, consider spending some of that money you made by selling your flat-screen TV to buy a self-help book on assertiveness, listen to a tape about standing up for yourself in a healthy manner, or get some short-term cognitive-behavioral therapy. Do whatever is necessary to transform yourself from a person who is passive and overly influenced or even dominated by others. You are a Good Woman with reasonable needs and wants. (If you weren't, you wouldn't have continued reading to this point in the book, I believe.) You deserve to live the life you desire. The American Geisha is kind and nonconfrontational as well as bold and assertive in pursuing what she needs and wants to be happy.

Stay Conscious of What You Need and Want

The Asian Geisha comes from an ancient culture that values contemplation, quiet time to escape the constant stimulation that seems to be so much a part of Western culture. It is during this quiet time that the Asian woman becomes aware of her deepest, most fundamental needs and desires.

Go to your quiet place, where you are alone and undisturbed in a relaxed situation, for thirty minutes minimum, with pen and paper. It could be in your home, at a coffee shop, in a library, somewhere in the woods, in a park, maybe at a bookstore. Do not be mindless, as I was. Instead, be thoughtful; gain an awareness of where you are now and of what you want for your future. Listen to your quiet self as you consider what your deepest needs are in a relationship with your Good Man. Write down your thoughts and feelings on a separate piece of paper. Fold the paper and keep it in this book for future reference. Return to that quiet place many times during the months ahead. Do some good thinking, contemplating, and experiencing of feelings. Write some of it down. Become conscious of what is important to you in a love relationship and marriage.

So many women think about their greatest relationship needs, then, in the heat of pursuit, they lose their focus and literally allow themselves to forget what they had earlier determined was important to them. That's what I did with Neil. The American Geisha does not forget but rather remains persistently focused on what she requires in order for her and her Good Man to be a happy, enthusiastic couple. You make business plans; you plan vacations. You had better, or else the business may founder and the vacation may be a disaster. Now it is time to plan for love and marriage—or else your desire for those things may founder and turn into a disaster, too.

See if you agree with this statement: "Probably nothing in my life will be as important to my happiness as being truly in love and married." I know it is true for me. If it is true for you, then doesn't it make sense to do whatever thinking and planning you can to help you find true love with a man who wants to marry you? Please say, "Yes, Older Sister."

While in your quiet space, please consider adopting Your Four Fundamental Needs as consciously chosen goals for your pursuit of the happy life you want. Of course, you may choose to *adapt* the Four Fundamental Needs, changing them so that they more perfectly support your own goals. As you contemplate your needs during different periods of your life, you may remove one or more goals from this list and add different ones of your own choosing. This is fine.

Find quiet time, lots of it. Think through what your most basic, nonnegotiable desires and needs are. Choose the fundamentals that reflect your true, unique self. Lastly, stay conscious of Your Four Fundamental Needs so that they serve as a vision to shape your actions as you move persistently toward your goals. To help you to stay conscious of Your Four Fundamental Needs, post them on the refrigerator, just to the right of the Four Core Characteristics of a Good Man.

Clarity of Purpose

Your hot, sexy, beautiful, feminine self must get organized in your pursuit of your Good Man. Developing a simple plan will transform the dreams and hopes you hold of love and marriage into *goals* that you can actually achieve, step-by-step, over the next year and a half or less. I know as your Older Sister how easy it is just to read this book without investing the time and effort to actually stop and write down a plan for attaining the happy, loving relationship you want. After all, I wasted eight long years without a plan. But, as your Older Sister, I have to tell you that by *not* having an explicit, written plan, you make it much more unlikely that my advice will lead you to love and marriage in a short time. Listen to me, please. I had no plan with Scott and Neil and wasted all those years. Then, while looking for the man who would become my husband, I had a plan, and it ended in my happy marriage twenty-one months after I began implementing it.

I promise I won't overdo it with my planning suggestions, but it is extremely practical and important to know what your priorities are and what you should do at different stages during your pursuit of love and marriage. Without a plan and goals, where would you wind up in eighteen months? I'll tell you where you'd wind up: in some *un*planned situation, and probably not in a loving marriage with a Good Man, perhaps not even on your way toward that loving marriage. Let Older Sister Py help you put together Your American Geisha Love and Marriage Plan.

On the other hand, if you have a plan, I promise that you will either have achieved your goals within eighteen months or that at the very least you'll be en route to those wonderful goals, perhaps just a little behind schedule. When you combine ongoing awareness with clearly stated goals, you make the world sit up and listen to you; you make things happen in your favor, according to your plans. You get what you want and need out of life by consciously and persistently pursuing whatever it is you desire. This clarity of purpose is key to the success of both the Asian Geisha in her pursuit of business and the American Geisha in her pursuit of love and marriage.

You need to spend a few minutes writing down your plan *now* (you can change it later, of course) in order to save you months or years of unfocused, wasted time in the *future*.

Characteristics of *Your* Good Man

In Chapter 7, we looked at the basics of what makes a Good Man. I hope you agree with me that the man you love and marry *must* have the following Four Core Characteristics:

1. He has good values.
2. He is aware and responsible.
3. He treats you well and is kind.
4. He is a happy person.

If you disagree with me about these four basic characteristics of a Good Man, now is the time to assert yourself. After all, this is *your* life, *your* Good Man, *your* plan.

Examine the list again. Cross out or change those characteristics you disagree with or do not consider absolutely necessary. Then, add to the list whatever additional absolutes you *definitely* must have as characteristics of your Good Man. Let me suggest the types of things you might consider adding:

- Age
- Height, weight
- Education level
- Income level
- Race preference
- Religious preference
- Type of job

- Has never been married
- Has no kids of his own
- __________________ (other)
- __________________ (other)

Let me add a caveat: I suggested in Chapter 7 that you keep your "absolutes" to a minimum, that you list only the most important, fundamental characteristics of a Good Man. I want to reemphasize that point here. Otherwise you could miss out on a really great guy simply because, for instance, he drives an old car. (My wonderful husband had *no* car when I met him, then he bought a 1970 [!] VW Bug shortly afterward.) So, try to be flexible about less important qualities such as income level and height; demand of your potential Good Man only the essential character traits that make him a good human being.

That said, if other characteristics are beyond your ability to compromise about, then add them to your list. You want to be practical, not merely theoretical, as you develop your plan. None of us—not you, not me—is perfect or perfectly accepting, so if your Good Man *must* meet certain standards of height or weight or intellect or religion or whatever, then go ahead and add those requirements. Try to keep your additional list short, but if he must, for instance, follow a certain religion, then write that down so that in your twelve-to-eighteen-month quest for love and marriage you don't "accidentally" wind up dating a man for a few days, weeks, months, or (ouch!) years whom, by your own definition, you could never marry.

Here are a few other qualities to consider (but you will probably not want to make these core requirements):

- Rich?
- Homeowner?
- Lives nearby?
- Sensitive?
- Good communicator?
- Good sense of humor?
- Handsome?
- Healthy?

- Sports nut?
- Loner? Gregarious?
- Family-oriented?
- Job-oriented (or not)?
- ___________________ (other)
- ___________________ (other)
- ___________________ (other)

If you have revised your Four Core Characteristics of a Good Man, replace the list that is posted on your refrigerator with your updated list. (Your Four Fundamental Needs are posted just to the right of your definition of a Good Man for you.)

Wedding (Getting Married) vs. Marriage (Staying Married)

Finally, as you create and implement your plan, always remember that ultimately you want a great *marriage* with your Good Man, not just a great *wedding.* Do not make getting married the focus of your efforts; rather, focus on the longer-term goal of *being* or *staying* happily married.

Never focus on the wedding itself. Do not let the wedding add psychological or financial pressure to your relationship. Do not let parents, family, or others influence the type of wedding you have. The wedding is important as a celebration of the event of your marriage, so it should be taken seriously as a significant life passage. Still, consider that yours should be smaller and less expensive rather than larger and more expensive.

As you focus on your relationship and on your long-term, happy marriage, you are more and more becoming an American Geisha.

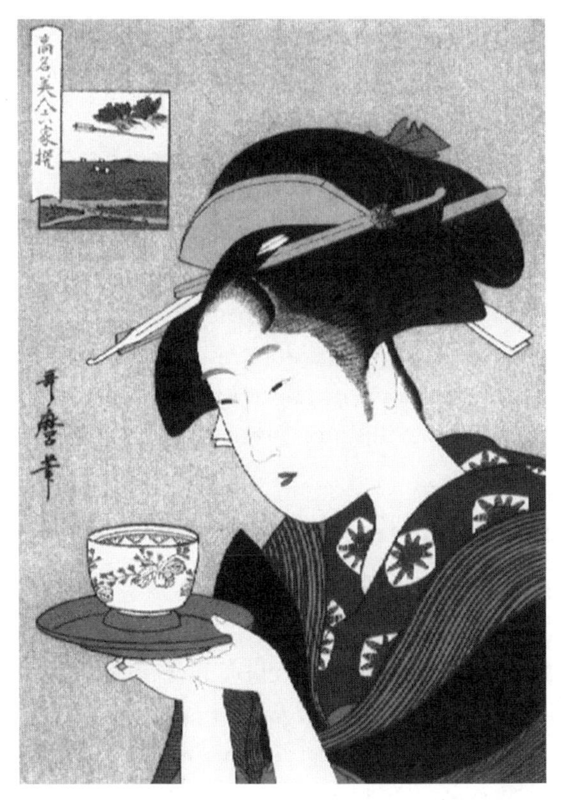

CHAPTER 9

A Plan to Achieve Your Best Weight — and Maintain It!

So far in this book I may have said some things, such as how much I love to fuck, that could be considered out of line. And some readers may feel that I ask you, as an American Geisha, to focus *too* much on taking good care of your man. Now, as I address the issue of body weight, I realize that the P.C. police will be ready to accuse me of all types of crimes against women, against feminists, and against heavy people. However, for my American Geisha Younger Sister to have her *best chance* of being married to her Good Man within twelve to eighteen months, I must gird myself for attack and carry on. I was in denial about my weight for a long time. I suffered such unhappiness, even after I faced the truth: I was fat, very fat. My fat was a major reason why men literally did not want to look at me or talk to me (or dance with me or date me or fall in love with me or marry me). They didn't want to get to know this nice, sweet, overweight woman.

Out-of-Control Weight and Its Impact

Throughout this book, as your Older Sister I have shared with you some of the mistakes I made, the lessons I learned, and the happy marriage that I finally achieved at age thirty-seven. I believe that *nothing* in all of my experiences and failures had a greater negative impact on me than my out-of-control weight. First, it had a direct negative impact on my confidence and happiness. What woman can be confident or happy when a man says to her face, as one did to mine, "You are a fat pig"? Or a female neighbor comments, "Your thighs are as big as my waist"? Or a brother half jokes that you're so round that if you fall down you would roll and not get hurt? Second, it had an indirect negative impact on me through the men whom I met. In a word, my being overweight was unfeminine. Men, being visual animals, were not attracted to me as a big woman. "Bigness" is masculine, not feminine. Most men are visually attracted to women who look feminine, who look relatively smaller in contrast to the man's relative bigness. The man's biological urge to conquer and protect, his testosterone-driven masculinity, is further engaged by your (relative) smallness and vulnerability. Even the Asian Geisha's whitened face, resembling that of a doll, suggests a vulnerability and fragility, a need to be protected. Let your best weight encourage your Good Man to feel that you are his delicate treasure, in need of his cherishing and protection.

Being overweight made me invisible to most men. At singles' dances men would stand over to the side and search the room with their eyes, deciding whom to ask to dance. I would watch them from afar and see that their glance wouldn't even slow down when it came to another large woman or to me. Their brains would barely register, "Big, keep moving," as their eyes continued to sweep around the room, pausing to look at the features of smaller women. Men literally never saw me, only saw the rather large space I occupied, and moved on. It hurt a lot that by the end of many evenings I had not said even a single word to one man. As nice as I was, no one at all had bothered to talk to me.

While I was dating Neil, I always felt hungry. I had to eat. But I now know that I was hungry for love and attention from Neil, not really for food. Over the five years I spent with him, I looked for excuses about why I needed to eat. Every food had some story attached to it. Even if I didn't have a reason for eating, I tried to make one up. It's a windy day; I need to have some hot soup. It's a full moon tonight; I must celebrate with rice cakes. I've got PMS; must have some chocolate cookies. I'm stressed; must get some protein from a pastrami sandwich or Italian sausage. I'm up early; I'll have a Deluxe Breakfast with hash browns at McDonald's. I heard that clam chowder was good for depression, so during a blue spell I ate the creamy soup daily for almost two weeks. Here was a favorite: When I missed being in Korea, I would go to L.A.'s Koreatown and overindulge in the good tastes of my old home. I was at my worst weight, just over 130 pounds (at four feet nine inches tall), while I was involved with Neil.

Attract More Good Men

If you are overweight, just a little or quite a lot, I want to help you, as I helped myself, to lose that excess weight and be both beautiful and more healthy. And more visible to more potential Good Men. If you are already married, you are already visible to your husband on a daily basis—or are you? Does it seem, perhaps, that he doesn't really notice you all that much, perhaps no longer expresses admiration for your body? Have you put on some pounds since the wedding, since the baby, over the years? If so, I want to help you make his eyes pay attention again, so that he will be newly attracted to his shapely American Geisha wife.

Most of the Good Men you might consider dating, having sex with, and marrying are attracted to lovely and feminine women who are at or near their most beautiful weight. An overweight woman, generally, is not considered either beautiful or feminine. Furthermore, being at your right weight is considered sexy, but being overweight is not. Yes, there are some men who find a large woman beautiful, feminine, and sexy (especially if she's toned herself nicely at the gym), but I think those numbers of men are relatively small.

The American Geisha's situation is at least as competitive as that of the Asian Geisha. Just as the Asian Geisha wants to present her best self to attract and keep clients, so do you, dear Younger Sister, want to present yourself at your very best to attract the attention of appropriate Good Men. You do not want to be invisible at the dance, in the office, at school, in the meeting, at the store, at the lake, or in the coffee shop. You want men who could be your Good Man to notice you in a positive way, to be struck by you, to be visually attracted to those things in you that men like about women: beauty, femininity, sexiness, and an appropriate, shapely body weight.

I feel that I can courageously throw this difficult topic of weight in your face because I've been there. I've suffered, as I know that right now some of you nice, sweet, overweight women are suffering. I say, let's suffer no more. Let's deny the truth no more. Let's put up with our overweight no more. Let's reach a beautiful weight and attract Good Men. Then let's choose one Good Man to marry, and let's get on with our incredibly happy lives. And let's do it now!

When you get to your most beautiful weight, you will automatically have an advantage in the competition for your Good Man. Why? Because at least 60 percent of other women are fat or obese and thus will likely be less attractive to most men. At your best weight you will not be invisible. Rather, you will draw his eyes to you because you will be so attractive.

Weight Matters

The Asian Geisha must be very aware and careful about her weight, for even after she is dressed in her several-layered kimono, she must appear slim, beautiful, and feminine to her rich male clients. Although the Asian Geisha is expected to drink much alcohol with the men she entertains, she does not eat at all while she works. Her lifestyle dictates that she eat when she arises around noon, then again at around 4:00 P.M., before she prepares for her evening, which begins at 6:00 P.M. When she returns home at midnight or later, she may have a snack before going to bed.

If she neglects her beauty, including her lovely figure, the Asian Geisha might well lose her rich businessmen clients to a slimmer, more beautiful geisha. Her competitive business demands that she always present herself at her best: beautiful and feminine, with a figure that pleases her clients' eyes.

Listen to what men told me about the importance of weight, especially as it relates to first attracting a man's interest:

"Body attraction is just as strong as, if not stronger than, facial."

"It's just initial physical attraction, nothing more."

"Usually the first impression is through someone's appearance."

"Young guys like a pretty face and a hot body."

"It takes a physical attraction to be interested in a woman."

"Most men are into looks only. Going on looks first is human nature."

"Men and women are definitely equal when it comes to how visual they are."

"The people who look the best are always the ones who have the easiest time finding partners to share life with. It has always been this way."

"Nowadays looks mean everything."

"I hear guys at work talking about women all the time, and the number-one thing you hear them say is, 'She is hot,' or, 'She is a dog.' It's all based on looks."

"I run away from overweight girls all the time."

"Procreation in itself is a quick process and only requires physical attraction. This urge and need is in all of us."

"Physical attributes are definitely something which draws me to somebody or would compel me to speak to (her)."

"While there is much more to a good relationship than physical aspects, the physical attraction is also a must for a relationship to last."

"Physical attraction is that crucial foot in the door.... Then you can learn more."

To a lesser degree, women also acknowledged the importance of physical attractiveness:

"Yes, it's true. Men are visual."

"A...man is turned off (by) an obese and unattractive woman. Being slim is a serious must."

"Men are always looking for the best-looking ladies to date. All they care about is a woman's look and hot body."

Early in my relationship with my husband, Rich, while I still weighed about 120 pounds, I asked him why he was dating me since all of his previous girlfriends had been thin. He said, "I see the nice shape of your legs." He didn't tell me that I was fat. Instead, he saw potential in my legs, which I thought were the worst parts of my body. He was telling me that if I could lose weight, then I could have nice legs. He bought me a bikini, even though my fat belly hung over the bottom piece. Rich motivated me even more to continue to lose weight. He always said to me, and continues to say today, "You get more beautiful every day."

Within two years I went from 130 pounds, alone, unhappy, unmotivated, always tired, and pessimistic, to 90 pounds, married, very happy, quite motivated, energized, and optimistic. Those 40 pounds that I lost mattered. My weight mattered. Without that weight loss I might still resemble the woman I described at the beginning of this paragraph, especially the "alone" and "unhappy" parts. I believe that *your* weight matters, too.

I don't really think I have to convince you too much that weight matters in attracting appropriate Good Men. What I do have to do is help you come up with a plan to lose the weight. Whether you are obese or twenty-five pounds overweight, or maybe just ten or fifteen pounds too heavy, I do have a plan for you—not a *diet* but a *plan.*

A Caution: Listen to Your Older Sister

Before your Older Sister describes her American Geisha Weight Loss and Maintenance Plan, I need to define some terms and issue a caution. If you are a bit too heavy or quite a bit too heavy, I want you to aim for a lower weight that will help you to present yourself at your best and most beautiful. The terminology I usually use to describe this target weight is "slim" or "your most beautiful weight." I do not want you to risk anorexia nervosa or bulimia by believing that you have to be reed-thin, "skinny," or "tiny" in order to attract your Good Man.

It is always a good idea to let your doctor know if you plan to lose weight, and to talk it over with her or him before you begin. Since I am not an expert in the fields of health, nutrition, diet, and exercise, I definitely encourage you to be cautious and safe, especially if you are quite overweight or obese. Of course, I learned my own lessons slowly, and lost my forty pounds without a doctor's supervision. And I did it despite friends and family who thought I was "getting too thin." People in your life get used to you at your heavier weight. They have a natural resistance to seeing you change, especially since your personality, attitude, happiness, and other traits are probably changing at the same time you are becoming thinner and more attractive. They prefer to relate to the old, familiar you, not this new, different you that they see emerging from your once-fat body. You may have to choose, as I did, to ignore some of the people who will say, "Oh, you look just fine the way that you are." But *do* consult with and listen to your doctor.

Let me put this in bold just to make the point as strongly as possible: **Do not seek to be skinny or too thin. And do consult with a physician if you plan to lose more than ten pounds.** Remember that you and I, Younger Sister, want you to be *healthy* when you marry your Good Man—both at a beautiful weight and healthy.

The American Geisha Weight Loss and Maintenance Plan

Oh, I'm getting excited. And I don't mean that my vaginal walls are sweating sexual lubricant. I mean I'm getting mentally excited at the mere prospect of writing these next paragraphs about a plan to help you get your weight under control and keep it under control. I feel so good to be at a beautiful weight (and to have stayed there for six years). I remember how bad I felt when I was fat. My excitement, though, is because I know that the American Geisha Weight Loss and Maintenance Plan (the "Geisha Plan") can work for you, too.

Notice that I wrote in the last sentence that the plan *can* work for you. I didn't write that it *will* work for you. Below, in bold type, appear two affirmations that I want you to read aloud enthusiastically and to believe totally. These statements, expressed sincerely and consistently, will begin to *guarantee* your success in reaching your most beautiful weight. Read them aloud:

- **I want more than anything to be in love with and married to a Good Man within twelve to eighteen months.**
- **I care more about love and marriage to a Good Man than I do about food.**

Right now, copy these two affirmations onto a piece of paper. It won't take long; they're short. Write neatly. Do it now! Thank you.

Now post the affirmations on your refrigerator, directly under the Four Core Characteristics of a Good Man that you posted after reading Chapter 7 and updated after reading Chapter 8. (My married readers will post revised affirmations, printed a few paragraphs down.) Now and for years after you have lost your excess weight and married the Good Man you love, you will keep these affirmations on the fridge as a reminder and an inspiration to continue to stay conscious of your desire to maintain a beautiful weight.

Four elements make up the American Geisha Weight Loss and Maintenance Plan. They are based on the above two affirmations. Here they are:

1. *You absolutely commit to your personal goal of marriage to the right man for you, and soon.* You are strongly motivated to do what is necessary to make

this happen, because love and marriage to your Good Man is a most important accomplishment in your life that will make you incredibly happy. (Ask yourself right now, "Is my American Geisha Older Sister right? Am I totally committed and motivated to being married?" Be honest, of course. Be aware of what you truly need and want.)

2. *You are personally responsible for prioritizing your needs and knowing that your need for love and marriage are higher priorities than your need for excessive food.* Put simply, you need love more than you need excess food. (Again, dear Younger Sister, ask yourself, "Do I truly value love and a great marriage over food? Is my heart with love or is my heart with food?")

If you have enthusiastically and excitedly answered both of my questions with a "Yes!" then the addition of two more factors will make your plan work today, tomorrow, next month, and even five or ten years into your great marriage:

3. *Stay aware and conscious of what your weight is and of what you're doing to lose or maintain weight by creating a weight/exercise chart and posting it on the refrigerator, right under your two affirmations.* (I'll tell you shortly what goes on the chart.)
4. *Lastly, find a photograph of you at your heaviest or at your current weight, and a photograph of you (no matter how young) when you were happy and comfortable with your weight.* I want you to stop reading right now. Mark this page. Then go find those two pictures. When you have the pictures in hand, come right back to this page and keep reading. (Please indulge your Older Sister, smile, and go get the pictures, now.) All right, you are back. You probably know what I want you to do with the two photos. Post them on the refrigerator, with magnets or scotch tape. The heavier picture goes above and to the left of your two affirmations, and the slimmer picture goes above and to the right of the affirmations. Again, your weight/exercise chart is posted under your affirmations, which in turn are posted beneath the Four Core Characteristics of a Good Man and Your Four Fundamental Needs.

For my married Younger Sisters or those in committed relationships, I suggest the following two, slightly revised affirmations. Read them aloud. Write them down on a piece of paper and post them on your fridge. (Of course, there's no need for you to post a list of the Four Core Characteristics of a Good Man. You already have your Good Man husband):

- **I want more than anything to revitalize my marriage (relationship), beginning now.**
- **I care more about love and my marriage (relationship) than I do about food.**

If you already have your Good Man, change numbers 1 and 2 of the Geisha Plan to:

1. *You are absolutely committed and strongly motivated to do whatever is necessary to revitalize your marriage (relationship), because an even better love relationship will make you incredibly happy.*
2. *You need a wonderful, improved marriage (relationship) more than you need excessive food.*

Numbers 3 and 4 are the same as for single Younger Sisters.

I would like for you to reread the four elements of the Geisha Plan and to be clear about what the plan entails. Please do it now. Once you've done that, I would like to simplify each of the four items, to make them easier to remember and thus more motivational. First, we can reduce each of the four parts of the Geisha Plan to a short sentence:

1. You are committed to getting married. (If you are married, you are committed to revitalizing your marriage.)
2. For you, love and marriage are a much higher priority than food.
3. You'll record and display your weight and exercise activities every day.
4. You'll add more beautiful pictures to the fridge as you lose weight.

Finally, we can simplify the Geisha Plan even more by reducing each sentence to its key word or concept:

1. Marriage (or revitalization)
2. Love

3. Awareness
4. Beauty

Personal Responsibility for Your Choices

By using the Geisha Plan to create *beauty* with the tool of *awareness,* you'll find *love* and *marriage.* And all the other good stuff, too: happiness, a Good Man, and a series of casual snapshots of you smiling more and more joyfully. A baby, too, if that is what you want.

Of course, I can't honestly make these guarantees to you, since only you can supply the commitment and motivation and inspiration to do what needs doing for the Geisha Plan to work. The Geisha Plan asks you to take a lot of personal responsibility for your choices:

- *You* are responsible to choose marriage (or to revitalize your marriage).
- *You* are responsible to choose to value love.
- *You* are responsible to choose to record your results daily.
- *You* are responsible to choose to become more beautiful.

Geisha Determination

Dear Younger Sister, the Asian Geisha has no one to guarantee her livelihood or to ensure that she'll attract more clients or find a good *danna.* The Asian Geisha is something like a sole proprietorship, with no one else to guarantee that all will go well. She can be a very tough, practical, determined businesswoman, not at all during the day the passive, obedient, "submissive" companion she becomes each night.

Sweet Younger Sister, you, too, must embrace this Geisha Determination, not in service to your business, of course, but in service to your happy marriage. Only *you* can guarantee that the Geisha Plan will work. Again, I have no choice but to tell you that you are responsible to choose to ensure your own success, just as the Asian Geisha is responsible for herself. You've chosen marriage, love, awareness, and beauty. Now choose again to guarantee that all of these things will happen.

It's always your choice. To read this book. To agree with me. To believe in the Geisha Plan. To reach your best weight and become more beautiful. It's always your choice. That's simply how life works, even with regard to weight and beauty. You make a choice. The American Geisha is happy that life works this way, because it is *empowering* to have choice. After all, *you* are responsible to choose, not someone else. You choose to be the right weight, to be beautiful, to be feminine. And then to do it. You become thinner, more beautiful, and more feminine. Responsibility and choice: Embrace them, dear Younger Sister. And become the shapely, beautiful, feminine woman you want to be.

As I wrote earlier, I'm all excited, bursting with enthusiasm and optimism. I hope you are, too. I hope you've been carried along by the wonderful possibility that beauty, love, and marriage will all come together for you because you've *chosen* to have these things in your life.

Earlier I wrote that I have a "plan" for you, not a "diet." I have no advice for you about carbohydrates, fats, proteins, caloric content of different foods, or what to eat. All of that comprises additional choices for you to make. The advice I have for you about food will be a few useful tips provided later in the chapter that you will choose to use or not.

The Geisha Plan is truly not a diet. Diets don't work very well. And if they do work at all, they tend only to work for a short time; then the weight returns. Did you notice that the four parts of the Geisha Plan say nothing about food, except that you care for love and marriage more than food? There are no menus or recipes. No calories-per-day goals, not even weight loss goals. There are only four parts to the Geisha Plan:

1. You are very committed to getting married (or to revitalizing your marriage), soon.
2. You are very motivated to find mutual love.
3. You will stay aware of your weight and exercise.
4. You are very motivated to be more beautiful.

Do you see "don't eat carbohydrates" anywhere in that list? No, of course not. Well then, Younger Sister, you might ask me, "How can I lose weight when you don't even help me to eat the right foods in the right amounts?" I have to answer by reminding you that you are not the average woman who wants to lose weight, picks a diet, crosses her fingers for luck, and hopes it will work. No, instead, you are an American Geisha Younger Sister who is different from the average woman. You are a woman who wants to be in love and married to a Good Man, and soon. You are a woman who has made this goal one of her very highest priorities. You have a Geisha Determination to succeed in your weight-loss goal, not only to help you be married soon but also to help you take the best care of your physical body.

"Sure," you might say to your Older Sister, "I want to be in love, married, beautiful, and healthy. But thousands of other women probably have felt similarly. Yet they're not able to lose weight, at least not permanently."

I would suggest to you that most women who diet are not as persistently conscious as you are of the strong connection between weight and finding (and keeping) beauty, love, and marriage. If they are less aware of that important connection, then they will be less determined than you to be successful in reaching their weight goals. You bought this book and have read this far. I *know* you are committed. I *know* you are motivated. I *know* you have a Geisha Determination to reach your most beautiful and healthy weight, then to attract your Good Man, fall in love, and marry. And to stay hot and sexy in the marriage. Now, read the next paragraph very carefully, Younger Sister.

The Key to Your Weight Loss Success: Awareness

There are four elements to the Geisha Plan: marriage, love, awareness, and beauty. I've suggested to you, dear Younger Sister, that weight loss can (will!) lead to beauty, then to love and marriage to your Good Man. The key to actually making all this happen is the third element of the Geisha Plan, awareness.

The daily chart you posted on the fridge is not for keeping track of the food or calories you consume. It is for keeping track of only two things: your lowest weight each day and exactly how much exercise you do each day. As simple as this is, it was the key to my weight loss and remains the key to my weight maintenance. By weighing yourself and recording your weight daily, you will never be surprised by a large weight gain, such as might happen if you weighed yourself only weekly. This is the key to your success: always being aware (consistently conscious) of your weight. I want you to be a loser—a loser of excess weight, a loser of weight as a negative issue for you, a loser of your poor body image. When you stay conscious of your weight on a daily basis, you will become the loser of whatever number of pounds you choose. Then you will become a winner in gaining control over your body.

Just as I do not suggest what you should eat, I do not suggest how you should exercise. By recording the exercise you've done on any given day (a blank in the chart meaning no exercise), you'll remain aware of your level of physical activity on a daily basis.

Set up your Weight and Exercise Chart as follows (this can easily be done in Word or Excel so that you can save the format and update the chart monthly):

- On an 8½ x 11-inch sheet of paper (use one sheet per month), create six columns.
- Across the top, label the columns:
  1. Day
  2. Date
  3. Weight
  4, 5, and 6. Fill in three specific exercises of your choice (for example, strength training, biking, stair-climbing, aerobics class, yoga video, brisk walking). Make sure you list activities you are likely to actually do. Or just write "exercise" in each of the three columns if there are many different activities you like to choose from.
- Under "Day," fill in Monday through Sunday, all the way down the page.
- Under "Date," type or write the corresponding date.
- Draw row lines across the paper, one per day.

Prepare several blank charts so that you have a chart ready to go when the new month starts.

Come up with a way to measure and record how much of each exercise you do. Current guidelines from various experts recommend getting forty-five minutes of moderately intense exercise at least five days a week (and not necessarily all at once), so one suggestion is to count each fifteen-minute "unit" of exercise you complete, since you have three spaces on your chart for exercise activity. If you attend an hour-long aerobics class, you've achieved a bonus fifteen minutes for the day! Another example: "hiking along the river at a brisk pace, thirty minutes." It counts for two of your three fifteen-minute units.

Awareness + Desire = Geisha Determination = Success

The life of the Asian Geisha has always demanded of its practitioners a strong sense of perseverance. First, the earliest phase consists of little more than being an observant maid in an *okiya* or geisha house. Then a girl must commit to years of training, followed by more years as an apprentice or Younger Sister. Finally she becomes a full-fledged geisha. I hold great respect for the successful Asian Geisha's commitment, persistence, and determination.

You, too, dear American Geisha Younger Sister, need that same Geisha Determination in order to do all that is necessary to accomplish your goal of a good marriage to a Good Man. Without determination it would be unlikely that most women could do all that is necessary to achieve their goals. My respect for your commitment to beauty, love, marriage, and awareness of your day-to-day progress is great.

Again, awareness truly is the key to your success. It is the foundation of all the other goals. That is why I had you post your two affirmations on the fridge, so you will look at them daily and stay aware of how important love and marriage are to you. I asked you to post your weight/exercise chart below the affirmations so you will record and look at your results daily and stay aware of how you are doing. And finally, I asked you to post your pictures above the affirmations, so that you may stay aware of how your new habits are making you more beautiful and healthy. (I still keep my weight and exercise chart up to date even after six years of marriage. Rich keeps one, too. And, yes, they are still posted on the fridge.)

That is all there is to it, my sweet Younger Sister. You do not need a specific diet to get to your most beautiful weight. Instead, what you need is great motivation...

...to have beauty, love, and a happy marriage

and

...to remain consistently conscious (aware) of how you are doing (specifically, recording daily weight and daily exercise) on your way to reaching your goal within twelve to eighteen months.

Based on your awareness of your daily weight and exercise and your great motivation to marry your Good Man, you will immediately adjust your intake of food or your output of exercise when the scale says you have gained weight or the exercise columns show two or three blank days in a row. When you are aware that your weight and exercise habits need adjusting, your great motivation won't let you accept the situation. Being aware of your power to choose, you will do the right thing. Older Sister trusts you.

Exercise and Eating Tips

Before I wrap up this chapter with a few helpful hints, I want to emphasize the element of awareness just one more time because it is so critically important to your weight loss success. If you stay aware of your weight and your exercise levels, you will be successful. Even if your weight and exercise results are not good for a day, still faithfully record the results. If, over a ten-day period, you gain seven pounds and do no exercise, continue to record your weight and exercise every day. Hey, no one is perfect. You'll have lapses. You'll occasionally backslide and get lazy. However, if you continue to stay conscious of both your weight and exercise, and continue to post monthly snapshots on the fridge, your great motivation to achieve beauty, love, and marriage will lead you to your goals.

Now, I'd like to leave you with a few tips for success. The Asian Geisha Younger Sister learns tips from her Older Sister by actually accompanying the Older Sister to work and observing firsthand how the Older Sister enters a room, converses with clients, offers to pour drinks, or bids good-bye. Dear Younger Sister, I was alone and without an Older Sister as I struggled to figure out how to lose weight and how to attract and to interact with men. Though I cannot be with you except in spirit, I want you to avoid struggle. I want you to enjoy becoming more beautiful, feminine, and healthy, and to enjoy the pursuit of and marriage to a Good Man.

If you are already married or in a committed relationship, let your partner know what you are doing about your exercise and eating, and seek his support. Let him know that his love and support inspire you to develop better exercise and eating habits.

EXERCISE TIPS

An exercise plan of whatever type (since it burns calories) is necessary to balance your eating plan of whatever type (since it supplies calories). Again, I am leaving it to you to determine both your specific exercise plan and your specific eating plan. Many books, classes, and videos are available to guide you. The American Geisha Plan only requires that you record your weight and the exercise activities you complete each day.

Exercise can make you feel so good. Rich and I live in a one-bedroom, 687-square-foot condominium. We exercise at home, using a workout bench, a stair-stepper, a sit-up machine, an electric jogging machine, a large exercise ball, two bicycles (kept on our patio), a pull-up bar, and a yoga mat for floor exercises, as well as various free weights. My point is you don't need much space to be able to exercise at home. Sure, it is cramped. But we are much better at exercising at home than we are at finding the time and motivation to drive to a gym. We're even a little bit proud that both our living room and bedroom seem more like "gym rooms." Consider investing in some exercise equipment you will enjoy using, even if it crowds the space you live in (you can find room for it). If you can develop a regular, consistent exercise regimen, and if you change it occasionally to keep it fresh and motivating, you'll take a major step toward achieving your most beautiful, ideal weight.

Exercise has been proven to produce pleasure-inducing endorphins in the brain, enhance mood, and boost confidence and self-esteem. It helps you overcome negative body image, aiding you in accepting and loving the body you have even as you sculpt yourself into the art piece that you want your body to become.

Here is a list of pointers for developing good exercise habits:

- At any time—perhaps at the end of each month—consider changing some of your exercises to help keep things fresh, new, and motivating.
- You have plenty of time to exercise. Do it instead of watching TV or overeating.
- Struggling with an urge to overeat? Go for a brisk walk instead.
- Difficult feelings? Don't eat—exercise! A vigorous workout like kickboxing is great for letting off steam and boosting mood, and yoga works well for reducing anxiety and learning to relax.
- Even a minute or two or three of free time can be turned into push-ups, sit-ups, stretching. Do it several times a day and your exercise chart will fill up with meaningful levels of activity.
- A study at Vanderbilt University, in Nashville, Tennessee, found that "hearty laughter" burned 160 calories per hour and boosted metabolism by as much as 20 percent, so watch sitcoms. I don't know that you could count it toward your daily exercise goals, but consider it a bonus.
- If you exercise consistently, you may be able to raise your resting metabolic rate, which can help you to burn more calories even when you are not exercising.
- Learn to love exercise for its own sake. When you make the choice to exercise, you gain feelings of control over your life, you feel better physically (more alert, more toned, more aware of your sexy animal body), and you feel better psychologically ("runner's high" isn't limited to runners but can be enjoyed by all exercisers). Plus you're taking a concrete step toward reaching your ideal weight, one of the goals in your plan to achieve beauty, love, and marriage within twelve to eighteen months. What's not to love about all that?

EATING TIPS

- Pick a weight loss goal of either five or ten pounds. When you reach and stay at that weight for a few weeks, choose another five- or ten-pound goal. Continue until you reach your most beautiful and healthy weight.

- Try any diet plan, if you like, but be aware that fad diets and those that are overly restrictive rarely work for the long term. People tend to gain weight once they go off them. Some diets even have attendant health risks. The best plan is to eat in a balanced, sensible way that restricts calories. Or don't follow any particular diet. Just be sure to record your weight and exercise activities each day.
- "Calories in, calories out"—You must understand that all diets obey a fundamental law of physics: If you take in *fewer* calories in a day than you burn (no matter whether the calories are in the form of carbohydrates, fats, or protein), you will *lose* weight that day. Conversely, take in *more* calories than you burn up, and you'll *gain* weight that day. It really is that simple. You must know and believe this basic truth. The difference between "calories in" and "calories out" dictates whether you lose or gain weight each day of your life, whether or not you are "on a diet." The only "diet" you need should be a combination of taking in fewer calories (by eating less) and burning up more calories (by exercising more and raising your metabolism). Forget everything else you've heard about diets. Just eat (somewhat) less and exercise (somewhat) more, and watch the pounds fall off of your frame, revealing a thinner, shapelier, sexier you. There are thirty-five hundred calories to one pound of body weight. So if you decrease your food intake by, for instance, fifteen hundred calories per week and increase your expenditure of energy by two thousand calories per week, you'll lose one pound per week. The laws of physics make that promise, not I.
- Get your "daily five" servings of fruits and vegetables. Although nutrition and diet experts don't always agree about the ratio of fat to protein to carbohydrate people should eat, one thing they all agree on is the necessity of consuming lots of fresh fruits and veggies. These so-called super foods contain loads of vitamins and minerals, health-boosting antioxidants, and natural sources of fiber. And, as a bonus, they help to fill you up while providing relatively few calories. Try eating a large green salad before dinner (with lemon juice

in place of fatty dressing, please), and you'll find it much easier to avoid overdoing it on the fried chicken or cheesy lasagna.

- The best time to weigh yourself is after you get up and use the bathroom in the morning, before you eat breakfast. You'll be at your lightest.
- If you wish, you may weigh yourself more than once a day. If you weigh less than you did previously, cross out the "old" weight for the day and write in the lower number. If you weigh more than previously, don't change anything on the chart. Record your lowest weight each day.
- When you are tempted to snack, first have a glass of water, plain tea, black coffee, chicken/beef bouillon, or a diet soft drink. A zero-calorie beverage may satisfy you for a bit and make you forget about food.
- Iced beverages and cold food burn calories because the body uses energy to raise the temperature of the drink or food to your body temperature (98.6° F). If you sleep in a cold room, you burn calories just to keep your body temperature stable.
- Learn to love black coffee or plain tea, with no sugar or milk. If you drink caffeinated coffee, tea, or diet soft drinks, limit your intake to a maximum of three servings per day.
- In the office, at home, or while out and about, only eat when you're seated in a chair. No eating on the sofa, in bed, while walking, or in the car.
- Don't engage in any other activities while you eat. No reading, working, watching TV, or surfing the Internet.
- Since we tend to finish whatever we see in front of us, including large portions, eat only in small portion sizes. Use a bread plate instead of a dinner plate when you serve yourself a meal. Eat whatever you like, but only half as much as you think you want. Super-size portions tend to be most Americans' biggest dietary downfall, so this is a very important tip.

- Relearn to pay attention to your body's satiety (fullness) signals. Wait to eat until you are truly hungry. Eat slowly. Then stop when you are satisfied, before you have stuffed yourself.
- Especially when you are out with others or on a date, eat more like a bird than a ravenous lioness. Be proud of your healthy, balanced eating habits.
- Watch out for problem snacking times, like midmorning or after work or between dinner and bedtime. Eliminate them entirely, or substitute a better snack, such as a piece of fresh fruit and a steaming cup of green tea for the pastry and coffee with cream and sugar you may now favor.
- If you are tempted into extra eating, try unloading your feelings in a journal rather than smothering their expression with inappropriate food. By learning to avoid eating as a way of dealing with your feelings, you gain the added benefit of becoming emotionally healthier.
- Eat fast food only as an infrequent treat, once every month or two. Watch the movie *Super Size Me* for motivation to stay clear of those places. Have you ever noticed that if you take the "s" out of "fast food," you have "fat food"? "Fast" food *is* "fat" food. Avoid it.
- Expect to be a little hungrier than you were when you ate too much, and endure some hunger proudly. Distract yourself. We all know the expression "No pain, no gain." More accurately for us, "No pain, no *loss*." Bear a little pain to be more beautiful. But don't overdo it. An eating plan that restricts calories too severely can lead to lowered metabolism (which you definitely *don't* want), mood swings, headaches, and reduced mental and physical performance in daily tasks.

Chances are that you will be dating before you have reached your most beautiful weight. If you meet and start dating a Good Man for you, let him know that you are working on losing weight. Tell him that now that you and he are dating, you are even more motivated to lose your excess weight so you can become more beautiful, feminine, and healthy for him and for yourself. When I was dating Rich, he congratulated me by saying, "You are a sculptor of the flesh, losing weight and revealing a more and more beautiful you." I have always liked that idea, that I am an artist re-creating myself as a more beautiful work of art. Earlier in the chapter I invited you to be a sculptor of the flesh and to create your own more beautiful self as you chip away the excess weight with new exercise and eating habits. Create the sexy you that makes you happy, proud, and more beautiful.

Remember the importance of awareness. Here's a quick review of the postings on your fridge:

- The Four Core Characteristics of a Good Man (at top; married American Geisha do not post this) and, immediately to the right, Your Four Fundamental Needs
- Pictures of you at your heaviest (on left) and your best (on right) weights
- Your two affirmations
- Your daily Weight and Exercise Chart (at the bottom)

As you choose to be beautiful, feminine, in love, and married within twelve to eighteen months, Younger Sister, I wish you the best and hope that you'll e-mail me and tell me of your successes in both losing weight and gaining your Good Man husband.

As you use your Weight and Exercise Chart, you are becoming a more and more beautiful American Geisha every day.

PART FOUR

★

Dating, Love, and Marriage

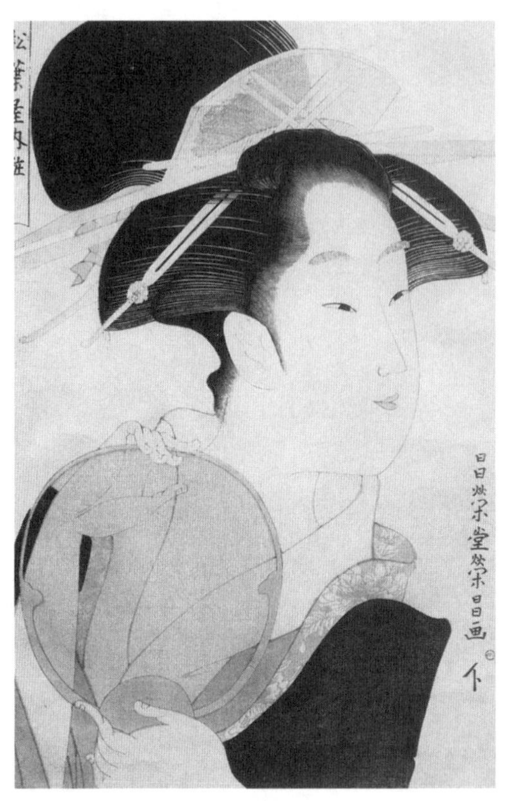

CHAPTER 10

Advance from Dating to Setting a Date

Let's review how far you have come as my Younger Sister American Geisha. You have adopted a Geisha Consciousness, recognizing the great yin power of your femininity in relation to a Good Man's yang masculinity. You are relaxed and confident of your worth and value as a Good Woman. You've fully explored your body and your sexual needs. You have begun to sculpt and tone your body and are on your way to achieving your most beautiful weight. You've increased your beauty by buying some new clothes, perhaps learning some new makeup techniques, and maybe having your hair styled. You've considered the characteristics you seek in your Good Man and defined your fundamental needs in a relationship. Now, after all of this preparation, you are ready to begin dating.

For you lucky ladies who are already married or in committed relationships, use this chapter to assess what you are doing to make your relationship even more loving and fulfilling. Single readers, use it to assess what you are doing in order to *get into* a happy, loving relationship with a Good Man.

The Art Gallery Opening

Wait. Is this book realistic and practical, as I promised you it would be? Are you so totally together that all you need to do now is to find a newspaper listing of this weekend's art gallery openings, slip on a little black dress, and go admire paintings on walls while you sip cheap merlot and subtly notice single male browsers, each with his own little plastic cup of wine? Perhaps. But, realistically, perhaps not. When I started dating again at age thirty-five, after breaking up with Neil, I certainly hadn't perfected my attitude, my sexual awareness, my weight, or my beauty. And most of my wardrobe still consisted of heavy Korean-made suits that my husband-to-be finally let me know were unstylish and, yes, unattractive on me.

Earlier, I encouraged my American Geisha trainee to go through quite a rigorous preparation before actually getting out there into the world of dating. It would be ideal if your personal confidence and attitude allowed you to be relaxed and calm. If you've fully explored your sexuality, perhaps even learning the skills of G-spot orgasm and female ejaculation, that's great. And you've lost all of the extra weight and toned your body. Fantastic. Yes, you've made yourself objectively beautiful. Fantastic again. And that little black dress is hardly lonely. You've invested in a new wardrobe. Wow. You are ready. Again, this would be ideal.

But what if you haven't yet reached that ideal? What if you are "working on it," but are not yet close to being there? I think this is probably the reality for most of us. We're "working on it." I know I was working on it (not always with a lot of awareness) when I reentered the dating scene in 1998. Sure, I would have been better off if I had worked on myself more before entering the singles pool. Yet life wasn't unfolding that way.

If, like mine, your life does not always unfold ideally, go ahead and jump into that singles pool anyway. Probably near the shallow end. Maybe just deep enough to get your feet wet. But do jump. I hope my suggestions have helped you to prepare yourself to be confident and strong when you begin dating. The stronger you are, the more likely your dating will be productive in a reasonable amount of time (twelve to eighteen months). But even if you are not perfectly prepared, go ahead and begin to get out and about. No matter your level of preparation, I hope you have been working continuously on the various elements that will strengthen you as you seek love and marriage with your Good Man.

The "Lucky Seven" Areas for Development

It is critical to continue to work consciously toward your ideal in the following seven areas. I call them the "Lucky Seven" because when you prepare yourself well in these areas, you will get lucky. That is, you will attract potential Good Men to you.

Is it truly luck? Hardly. There is great truth in the saying that luck comes to those who prepare to be lucky. Without the preparation, there is probably little luck. With full or ideal preparation, you'll be able to choose from among several (or even many) potential Good Men.

Let's quickly review the Lucky Seven development areas:

1. To be positive, optimistic, and happy
2. To be relaxed, at ease, and confident (not desperate)
3. To be sexually aware of your desires and capabilities

4. To be at your most beautiful weight
5. To be fit, toned, and healthy
6. To be beautiful, feminine, and sexy (Geisha Attractiveness)
7. To be dressed well (including makeup, if that's part of your personal style)

If you, dear Younger Sister, have approximated your own ideals in these areas, then I feel confident—and you should too—that you will be married to your Good Man in twelve to eighteen months. On the other hand, if you jumped into the dating pool early, before fulfilling your potential, then you should be committed to continuing to work consistently on each of these areas, and you can expect that it will take longer to reach your goal of being happily married. It takes real work and effort to be married to your Good Man in a fairly short time. If the work is done more slowly, expect the result to be achieved more slowly.

I took too long (*years* too long!) to realize the power that I would have to attract potential Good Men by being positive and happy instead of depressed. By being relaxed and confident instead of desperate. By being sexually aware instead of naïve. By being slim and trim instead of obese. By being toned and healthy instead of out of shape and unhealthy. By being beautiful, feminine, and sexy instead of plain and aggressive. And by being well dressed instead of not caring about how I dressed. (Oh, how it hurts to write and to face these truths, even now.) What *was* I thinking? I wanted to have good relationships with men and to get married, but I kept myself in a condition that I now realize very few men (and, as it turned out, not Good Men for me) would be attracted to.

If You Have Achieved Your Goals

I'll assume that, motivated both by reading *Sex Secrets of an American Geisha* and by your strong desire to marry your Good Man, you have developed sufficient inspiration to achieve your goals in the Lucky Seven areas. If you have, in fact, already achieved what you set out to do in each of these areas, your Older Sister wants to congratulate you enthusiastically. Yet I still give you advice similar to what I offer American Geisha in training who have not yet reached all of their goals:

- Stay aware of your progress in each of the Lucky Seven areas.
- Continue improving yourself in each area.
- Avoid carelessly backsliding from the progress you have attained.

The Lucky Seven Chart

Whether or not you've achieved the Lucky Seven ideals, you need to stay aware of and continue to work on each area, either to maintain or to strengthen your position. I want you to record in the following chart how you're doing, both right now and again just before you enter the dating pool. Your awareness of where you are now and your taking responsibility for getting to where you want to be are critically important to being married to your Good Man in the shortest time possible.

By now you've read nine full chapters, well over half of the book. So take a few minutes to think about your progress. Perhaps thumb back through the earlier chapters. If you're keeping a journal, reread what you've written there. Then write down in the chart on the facing page a number between one (much work to do) and ten (achieved your ideal) for each area. Remember that when you have prepared yourself in these seven areas, the "luck" of your good preparation will help you to find and to marry your Good Man, soon.

Once you have assessed where you stand in the Lucky Seven development areas, you have a baseline or starting point that you can compare against your later assessments. These assessments are not so much to grade you but rather to keep you aware of these important areas and, over time, to help you see your continuing progress in each area. What is most important about this chart is seeing for yourself that you are moving, no matter at what pace, toward your goals. As long as you are progressing toward your ideals in the Lucky Seven development areas, you are moving closer and closer to the day when you will marry your Good Man.

Notice that the second column is for a reassessment just as you are about to dive (or step cautiously) into the dating pool. I want you to see

THE LUCKY SEVEN DEVELOPMENT AREAS

Use a 10-point rating scale, where 10 = "I've reached my goal/ideal" and 1 = "I still must work hard on reaching my ideal." Be honest with, but not too hard on, yourself. Use the results to stay *aware of* and *responsible for* the goals you desire.

Development areas	Now (as you read this book)	Just before beginning to date	After 3 months of active dating	After 6 months of active dating
1. Positive attitude				
2. Relaxed confidence				
3. Sexuality				
4. Ideal weight				
5. Fit and healthy				
6. Beautiful, feminine, and sexy				
7. Clothes and makeup				

progress between the far lefthand column ("Now") and the second column ("Just before beginning to date"). Record additional assessments (and ongoing improvement) in the final columns three months after you begin dating and then again six months after you begin dating. When you reach your ideal in any area (a score of 10), the chart will help you see that you are maintaining it.

(All of the Lucky Seven areas are equally important whether you are married or single. For that reason I want my married American Geisha, and those in committed relationships, to record where you are when you first read this chapter, and again three, six, and nine months later. Accordingly, those readers can cross out the headings in the last three columns and write in "3 months later," "6 months later," and "9 months later.")

To enhance your awareness of your status in each area, post a photocopy of this chart on your refrigerator, just to the right of your weight and exercise chart. Remember, do not be hard on yourself in your judgments. Just be sure you stay conscious of your progress by doing the three follow-up assessments after your initial one. Your refrigerator will be happy to know that this is the last item I will ask you to post there, except for the monthly snapshots, which will continue forever (and which you can proudly spread all over the fridge).

Be Different from—and Better than—Other Women

The Asian Geisha competes against hundreds of other geisha to win the business of her clients and to be asked back repeatedly to different teahouses and events. She does this by distinguishing herself from the other geisha as much as she can. She seeks to be somewhat different from and better than the others. Perhaps more beautiful. A better conversationalist. A better dancer or musician. More humorous. More polite or daintier. More girlish. Smarter. Better dressed or made-up. A nicer smile. More personable. More effusive. Prettier and more interesting kimonos. She always wants to learn to do whatever might give greater pleasure to her clients than her competitors give.

In fact, she will probably continue her schooling and take various classes throughout her career, always trying to become a better geisha. Actually, the Asian Geisha doesn't have to learn to *do* (dance, play music, conduct a tea ceremony, sing) as much as she has to learn to *be*. For much of her time as a geisha, she will be in the company of groups of men who actually may not interact very much with her. She may simply stand, sit, or kneel, be calm and attentive, appear happy, and be both beautiful and beautifully dressed. In summary, much of her time is spent not doing anything, but rather just being very feminine (there's that word again). If she is seen as different from and better than other geisha at simply being very feminine, she will probably have happy clients and a long, successful career.

You, too, dear Younger Sister, must seek to be different from and better than your competition in the dating world, where there are lots of other women that a Good Man might ask out instead of you. It is a fact that you have lots of competition, especially for the relatively few really Good Men out there, one of whom might someday become your husband. That is why you must do all you can to distinguish yourself from the other women who are your competition.

Pardon me for reminding you, Younger Sister, but you are looking for a pretty incredible guy. I'll bet the Good Man you seek is one with all or most of the characteristics I've encouraged you to seek, plus any more requirements you may have added to your list of the Four Core Characteristics. This man you want for a husband can himself be pretty choosy about whom he wishes to date and to marry. That's the reality: He's a good catch. For you to be the one who catches him, you have to be a pretty good (great!) catch, too. You need to be different from and better than all the other women that your potential Good Man is exposed to in his search for his potential Good Woman, you! If you are to overcome all of the competition and win your incredible Good Man, it will be because you are an incredible Good Woman. Since the admission standards to your vagina and to marriage with you are tougher than Harvard University's entrance requirements, you must expect that you too should be of the highest possible quality.

Your Older Sister is not going to tell you specifically how and where to go to meet men. (But I will list some possible ways to meet them; see below.) I do, however, wish to suggest that you do not want to meet just *any* men, but rather only *appropriate* men for you. I hope you did a little work back in Chapters 7 and 8, where we discussed requirements for someone to qualify as a Good Man for you. With that work done, you have a good idea of the type of man you seek.

In getting into the dating scene you want to meet a large number of possibly appropriate men, so that you have several (or many) men to choose from when deciding whom to date. If someone you meet is obviously or even intuitively not a Good Man for you (for whatever reason), do not date him. Try to get to know a man a little before you accept a date so that you do not inadvertently date an inappropriate man and wind up wasting your (and his) time.

Your Older Sister knows that it is often hard to ascertain a man's appropriateness before accepting a date with him. But sometimes you have enough information about him to cause your intuition to indicate either "possibly appropriate" or "probably inappropriate." Listen to and trust your intuition. It is your subconscious trying to make you conscious of your deeper knowing about any given situation. You can also follow the advice I offer later in this chapter (in the section "The American Geisha Must Be Selective") for helping you to determine whether to pursue a dating relationship with any particular man.

Now That You Are Dating

You are out there, dating, whether or not you are fully and ideally prepared. Congratulations, dear Younger Sister. You are making yourself available to potential Good Men who might see or hear of you and be attracted to you. I hope that you are feeling confident, positive, and optimistic about your journey to love and marriage. You are focused and aware of becoming more beautiful, feminine, and sexy every day. Your weight is changing for the better (or staying near its best), and you exercise regularly. Your health is good or improving. You know you are a hot, sexy lady. Your wardrobe gets more attractive each month. Even your makeup and hairstyle are more flattering. You are an artist of the flesh who has created and sculpted a beautiful, feminine, and sexy woman of yourself. Now you proudly and happily and *with a sense of fun* set off on your twelve- to eighteen-month journey to love and marriage.

I am so happy if you are leaving your home two or three evenings a week to open yourself up to the possibility of meeting appropriate men. Don't think that I want you out there seven days a week, doggedly pursuing your Good Man. Wouldn't that seem a bit desperate? I think so. You want to be relaxed, happy, and having fun, not so focused on men that there is nothing else in your life.

In fact, I want to suggest two things, Younger Sister, that should remain in your life both now, as you date, and later, after you are married. The two are hobbies and girlfriends. A hobby or an interest (or interests that change over time) gives you outlets for your passion. Do not give up all your hobbies to pursue your Good Man. Let him know that you have other interests. Mine are (or were) papermaking, collage, beading, writing poetry, candle-making, scrapbooking, knitting, soapmaking, gardening, furniture painting, rubber stamping, hand bookmaking, and writing articles for magazines.

Find your own interests and pursue them while dating and after marriage so that both you and your man know that you have a life beyond the relationship. You want to present yourself as a whole woman, as someone with interests in the outside world, not as a woman solely focused on men and relationships. You are more interesting (more attractive) to a man when he senses your depth and distinct personality. This makes you different from (and better than) so many other women with narrow focuses.

Always maintain active relationships with your girlfriends, if for no other reason than to give your partner a little relief from being the only one you talk to. The men in your life will appreciate that your girlfriends contribute to making you happy in ways that a male simply cannot. And every Good Man knows that a happy wife is going to make him happy, and that when both of you are happy, you will have a happy relationship.

Where to Meet Potential Good Men

I wrote earlier that I would not recommend specific ways to meet men. But I do want to encourage you to consider exactly how you might put yourself in a situation where you could meet or run into an appropriate man, a potential Good Man, a possible future husband. Here is a long but not totally inclusive list to stimulate you to consider how many different ways are open to you. Of course, you'll think of even more.

- Through a family member
- Through a friend
- At a singles party or event
- At school
- At a reunion party
- At work
- At the supermarket
- At the gas station

- At the beach or lake
- At your gym
- On a hike
- On an airplane
- At an airport
- At a dance
- While jogging or walking
- While biking or roller-blading
- While skiing or snowboarding
- On vacation
- On a cruise
- On a bus
- While walking your dog
- In a coffee shop
- In a donut shop
- In a bar
- In a karaoke bar
- In the library
- In a bookstore
- At a street fair
- At a networking event
- At an alumni event
- At a garage sale
- At the laundromat
- While visiting a client
- At a business-training event
- At a conference
- In a business meeting
- At the annual company picnic or holiday party
- At a job site

- At breakfast, lunch, or dinner
- In the company or school cafeteria
- At your condo or townhouse homeowners' meeting
- At your apartment swimming pool
- In an elevator
- Walking in your neighborhood
- At a religious event
- Through politics
- At a book-signing event
- At a Toastmasters group or other club
- Through a public-service project
- At a fundraising event
- At volunteer organizations
- On the Internet
- Through a dating service
- On a blind date
- At a holiday event (e.g., fireworks on July 4th)
- At a wedding or reception
- At a sporting event
- On a company-sponsored sports team
- At a car wash
- In a bank or movie line
- Inside the movie theater
- While speed-dating
- Through a personal ad in a local weekly newspaper
- At a computer (or other) class
- On a golf course
- At a bowling alley or tennis court
- At a comedy club
- At a music concert

- At an art gallery opening
- At a museum event
- At a play, during intermission
- In the rain or snow
- While window shopping
- While shopping at a mall
- At a hobby shop (shared interest)
- At an open-mike night
- At a farmers' market
- At a nightclub
- At a restaurant (especially a buffet)
- At a wine tasting
- In a fast-food line

I'd like to know where you met *your* Good Man. Please e-mail me.

The American Geisha Must Be Selective

The Asian Geisha may meet a potential new client by being approached directly by an individual or an organization wishing to have her attend a private function. Or, more commonly, she may be approached through her own *okiya* (geisha house) or through the geisha-booking service in her district. In each case she has final say as to whether she chooses to attend any given function. If she attends inappropriate functions (for instance, at a less respected, less prestigious teahouse), other potential good clients may bypass her because of her tarnished image. Thus, the Asian Geisha has to be selective about which events she chooses to attend.

You, dear Younger Sister, must also choose carefully from among the men you attract. You waste time dating a man who has little or no potential to be a Good Man for you. Not only that, but your image may suffer from dating inappropriate men, perhaps discouraging other men from getting to know you, possibly including a man who may have been right for you.

No matter how you've met a man, the first thing you want to do is try to ascertain whether he has the potential to be a Good Man for you. If he seems to have that potential, you certainly would be open to seeing him further. If he seems not to have that potential, it is best not to see him further, unless seeing him further would open good social networking opportunities for you. Remember always to be frank and honest and nonmanipulative and kind to the men you encounter while dating. Don't lead on an inappropriate man once you realize he is not a candidate for a longer-term relationship with you.

Let's say that a man you meet at a bookstore coffee shop asks you out for dinner. According to whether or not he seems to have some Good Man potential, you could answer him in one of several ways.

SITUATION 1: NO POTENTIAL

If you judge quickly (or after a forty-five-minute chat) that there is either no potential or so little potential that you do not want to invest any further time, you want to discourage him. You might respond, "Thank you, that's sweet of you. But I can't." If he persists (which he probably won't), say truthfully, "I'm just not available right now. It's been nice to meet and to talk with you." Do not touch him and do not be your most fun, likable self. After all, you want to discourage him.

SITUATION 2: POSSIBLE POTENTIAL

If you sense some potential but are unsure, you want to be somewhat neutral. You might say, "Thank you, that's nice of you. But why don't we just have coffee again? Maybe on Friday, right here. How's that for now?" After your second chat over coffee, perhaps you'll know more clearly whether to end this budding relationship or to allow it to proceed to a real date (lunch or dinner). Maybe touch his arm or body in some casual way. Let him see some of your warmth.

SITUATION 3: DEFINITE POTENTIAL

When you sense that he has some real potential to be a Good Man for you, you want to encourage him. Accept his invitation. Perhaps say, "Thank you. That sounds lovely/wonderful/nice/like fun. I'd love to/like to." As you plan the details of your date, be sure to consider your physical safety by arranging to meet in a public place with you driving your own car. Lunch rather than dinner may feel more comfortable. As you sense this potential (and before he asks you out), touch him, lean toward him, sit closer. Let him get a good sense of your happy self. These actions encourage him. Unbroken eye-to-eye contact also shows your interest.

In your first meeting it is usually inappropriate to bring up any part of your life plans and goals (including marriage or kids). Consider getting into this subject area during your second get-together, whether it is over coffee or a "real" date. This is not to put immediate pressure on the man but to honestly show him who you are while also asking him about his own life plans.

Whenever you talk to a date or boyfriend (a man who is not yet your fiancé) about such things as marriage or kids, do not pressure him by saying, "If I marry you...," or, "If we had kids...." Avoid using him as the example. Simply let him know your general, long-range plans. Say, "I plan to marry in the future," or, "I'll have kids someday."

You've Decided to Date Him. Now What?

You have decided that a man who has shown you some attention should be encouraged because he seems to be a Good Man based on what you know of him. Though who can be sure until you date him for a while?

One of your goals is to meet and date Good Men, so you are likely to be receptive to any suggestion he might propose, such as lunch or dinner or coffee or a drink or a ride home or a shared taxi or even a suggestion that "we should do something sometime." Perhaps you had interest in him before he did in you, and you put yourself in positions where you saw or spoke to each other. Your confident belief in your Geisha Attractiveness lets you know that you have made yourself very appealing. There is a good chance he'll be attracted to you if he is simply in your presence often enough to notice you. Once noticed, you have a confidence that all you need to do is "be," and he'll "do" what is necessary to move the relationship forward. You have done what was necessary to get him to notice you (oh so feminine), but you don't pursue him by approaching him or by asking him out. You arrange things so that he can be direct (oh so masculine) and approach you first.

If there is no one of any particular interest to you at the moment, then you need to do the things that get you into the presence of potential Good Men. You must commit to leaving your home fairly frequently to enhance your chances of meeting someone. This is a critically important step in the meet-date-marry process. You can't meet someone if you're at home in your bathrobe, idly watching TV, half-interestedly stroking your vulval lips through your panties while you think about what you'll wear to work tomorrow.

An Asian Geisha would starve if she stayed home all night since her business hours are from 6:00 P.M. to 2:00 A.M. Although she may have clients with whom she has ongoing relationships, she also attends functions that are somewhat like blind dates since she may have little idea of what to expect from a new client or a new teahouse until she actually shows up for the event.

Although a blind date may not work out for either the Asian Geisha or the American Geisha, each is happy to have attracted the attention. Each is optimistic that out of any of the ways in which she might meet a prospective client or Good Man, something good could happen. Of course, her happy attitude only increases the chances that she will connect positively with the men she meets.

You have to take a chance and get into circulation. The word "circulation" brings to mind the veins and arteries that circulate the blood. If you, dear Younger Sister, represent a single drop of blood, then to get into the circulatory system and to mix with tens of thousands of other drops means you're going to have to jump from the sidelines into a vein or artery. Go ahead. Get out there! Get into circulation! Mix with all of those other "single" blood drops. One of them is your Good Blood Drop. Otherwise, you will be "out of circulation," out of touch, unreachable by the Good Men you want to meet. This must not happen. Get out. Leave your home. Circulate.

In the West, traditional business hours are from nine to five. I want you to think of the Asian Geisha's business hours, 6:00 P.M. to 2:00 A.M., as your *personal* hours. It is during these hours that you will need to get out and about, to increase your exposure to men. The Asian Geisha goes to parties and other functions every night, often seven days a week. She is disciplined. Even if she doesn't feel like it one particular evening, she applies her makeup, fixes her hair, calls her dresser to come over, and goes out anyway, with a smile on her face.

You probably will not go out seven days a week. But you, too, must have discipline, my dear Younger Sister. You must circulate so you can allow yourself to be discovered by a potential Good Man. Sit at your vanity table and apply your makeup. Fix your hair. Select your clothes from your carefully chosen wardrobe. Then go out, alone or with others, with a happy smile on your face and an optimistic attitude in your heart. Know that you are doing the right thing to help you achieve the most important goal in your life: to find a Good Man, to fall mutually in love, and to marry.

From Dating to Dating with Sex

You have prepared yourself for the dating world. You have gotten out and have attracted some potentially Good Men, one or more of whom you have chosen to date. Now (or eventually) you must deal with the question of whether or not to have sex with a potential Good Man.

(Some of you, for whatever personal reasons, will choose not to have sex with anyone until you are married or at least engaged. I certainly understand and respect your choice. This section is for women who would consider having sex while dating.)

The key to deciding whether to have sex with a specific man is first to determine that he is basically a Good Man and that he is possibly willing to meet the Four Fundamental Needs that we discussed in Chapter 8. You definitely want to avoid having sex at *any* time with *any* man who is *not* a Good Man.

The Asian Geisha's regular clients are nearly all quite wealthy men. Were they to learn that she was having sex with a man of lower stature (an inappropriate man), her reputation and value would diminish and previous clients might stop engaging her services. As an American Geisha, Younger Sister, it is very important that your value stay high to prospective Good

Men. Both the Asian and American Geisha try always to keep a smile on their faces and to maintain the positive attitude that serves them well. Your Older Sister, your American Geisha trainer, needs just for a moment to deal with some less than positive aspects of having sex with someone who is not a Good Man for you. You waste time. You waste emotions. You waste energy and perhaps money. You lose your focus. You run the risk of pregnancy, sexually transmitted diseases, psychological upset. Wow! All for a Wrong Man. No geisha, Asian or American, would respect herself or be respected for such behavior. Image is so important to the Asian Geisha. In a sense, if her image of class and selectivity is destroyed, there is nothing left. To be an Asian Geisha is *all* about image.

You, my dear American Geisha, are much more than simply an image; you are a Good Woman of substance and worth. Though you are my Younger Sister and not a fully trained American Geisha, you are still too intelligent and classy to dawdle with a man you know is not right for you. You will be as kind to him as you can as you terminate the relationship, and you will move on in a timely manner. And you will not have sex with him.

Many men see the Asian Geisha as among the hottest, most beautiful of all women, yet she is extremely selective about the relatively few men she takes to her bed. If she were not, her image could be damaged and her business dry up, for she might be perceived as more of a concubine than a geisha.

The Asian secret the American Geisha learns is that although she is always hot and sexy, this does not translate into being *sexual* with a man until she has ascertained that he is basically a Good Man for her. The American Geisha takes a businesslike attitude toward sexuality that is similar to the Asian Geisha's. If she is sexual only with the relatively few Good Men she meets, her image to other prospective Good Men remains positive, classy, and selective; she is hard to win but worth it. Truly, the choosy American Geisha is more valuable and more attractive to other prospective Good Men. She knows what she wants in the long term. She wants to be sexual only with a prospective Good Man who might be a candidate for a committed relationship. Determine what Your Four Fundamental Needs are and how likely it is that this Good Man could be the one to fulfill them.

Sex Before Commitment

You may imagine that agreeing to have sex before you have a monogamous commitment from a man could lead to the commitment you seek. Wrong. If he gets to have sex with you before commitment, you lose some of your power to get him to commit. After all, why should he commit further if he's already having sex with you? Yes, you may answer, but with sexual intimacy he'll fall for me even more. Wrong again. With sexual intimacy before commitment, all you know is that his cock is in love with your vagina. You are beautiful, feminine, and have a gorgeous, fully shaved vagina. Of course he's in love with your vagina! What man wouldn't be? But you want his love for *you* to come before his love for your sexual organs. My husband loves me (and tells me) and loves my cunt (oops!) and tells me. But he had to like and love and commit *to me* first, before he got to experience my vagina, which he instantly loved, too.

Remember, just as the Asian Geisha, "those classiest and most exclusive of women,"[1] receives a substantial commitment (including a marriagelike ceremony and a financial commitment) before she gives herself sexually to her *danna,* an American Geisha must gain a Good Man's commitment before he gains entrance to her beautiful vagina. By the way, "instant commitments" don't count. If you've teased him to the point of nakedness or of being only an undergarment away from nakedness, and then ask him, "You do love me, don't you?" do not be fooled by the answer "Of course I do." That is his cock talking. At this point his brain has been kidnapped by his throbbing cock. All his brain blood now resides in his swollen cock, and his cock is totally in charge of what his mouth says. "Of course I love you" means "Of course I love your vagina." If you let a Good Man fuck you before commitment, you risk losing that Good Man because you were too easy; you weren't selective or demanding enough. Be patient. Get the commitment first. Your hot, wet vagina needs to be fucked only by a *committed* Good Man.

It may take you several weeks or several months of dating a man to determine whether you want to have sex with him. This is not an unreasonable time frame for such an important decision. Again, it is totally appropriate to share your thoughts with a man regarding your qualifications of a Good Man and Your Four Fundamental Needs. It is even reasonable to give him a copy of this book so that he understands what will lead to your decision. Also discuss how he sees your relationship, both now and in the future. If you decide that sex with this man is appropriate for you, then mutually commit to monogamy and go for it. If he is unwilling to commit to monogamy, do not agree to have sex with him. (Remember: Before having sex, mutually disclose your sexual histories, get tested together, and guard against pregnancy. More on this can be found in Chapter 11.)

If you realize over time that this relationship shouldn't lead to sex, then you must stop dating him. Even if he is a Good Man, you may decide that he is still not someone you want to have sex with, probably because he cannot fulfill all of your Fundamental Needs. Be kind and gentle as you end the relationship. But be resolute. You need to move on, learn whatever lessons are there for you, and get back into circulation.

You Are Dating with Sex. Now What?

Always keep in mind your very reasonable goal: You want to be mutually in love and married within twelve to eighteen months. You told this man your goals before you started having sex with him. You'll continue to remind him occasionally of your goals now that you have deepened your intimacy by engaging in monogamous sex.

Both before you have decided to have sex with him and after you start to have sex with him, it is key to moving your relationship forward toward engagement and marriage that you tell him this: Your heart and body are capable of greater and greater commitment to him as you experience his greater and greater commitment to you and to the relationship.

If he has not proposed marriage to you of his own initiative, there will come a time (sooner rather than later) when you will have to remind your Good Man again of Your Four Fundamental Needs, including marriage (assuming that marriage is what you want at this time in your life). Without nagging or manipulation, but with the confidence and assertiveness of someone who knows she is a Good Woman worthy of having what she reasonably wants from life, you will assertively pursue marriage with this Good Man. You will encourage him to decide whether he wishes to marry you. And if, in your judgment, he puts off such a decision too long, you will lovingly tell him that you cannot wait beyond a specific date for him to decide, set a wedding date, and buy an engagement ring. I suggest allowing him one to two months from when you bring up the deadline. (Some of you—and some of your Good Men—may find twelve to eighteen months too short a time to know someone well enough to commit to marriage. If it seems too short to you, adjust the timeframe to your preference.)

If he still can't decide, or if he decides not to marry you, stop seeing him. Tell him that you love him but you need marriage. Tell him you must move on, that he is a Good Man, but just not *the* Good Man for you, since he does not want to marry you. If he says he loves you, tell him, "You may love me, but if you do not love me enough to marry me, I must move on." Add, if it's true, "I love you, too. But it's not enough. I want to be married." Tell him to be in touch again only if he decides he wants to marry you.

Immediately start dating other people, but hold off on having any sexual relations for at least two months. He may miss you so much over those two months that he comes to you with a ring and a wedding date. If he doesn't, then learn from your time with him, shed some tears if necessary, and move on to being totally open to meeting the Good Man who *will* want to marry you.

A reminder: Once you're engaged, with a ring and a wedding date, do not totally focus on the wedding. As I mentioned in Chapter 8, what should be important to you is your *relationship,* now and over the many happy years of your marriage. You are more and more becoming an American Geisha when you focus on the great relationship between a Good Woman and her Good Man.

CHAPTER NOTE

1. Leslie Downer, *Women of the Pleasure Quarters* (New York: Broadway Books, 2002), 260.

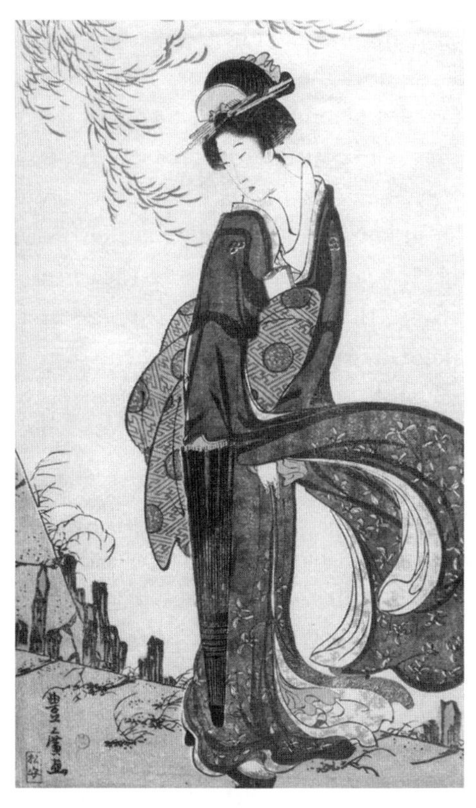

Chapter 11

"I Could Only Do That for My Husband"

The Asian Geisha's profession involves teasing her clients with her skills (dance, musical instruments, conversation), her focused attention, her beauty, her femininity, and her sexuality. Very rarely, and not at all for most of her clients, does she provide any kind of sexual experience.

She saves the greatest commitment of her attention, time, and sexuality for only one man, her *danna,* or sponsor/patron. A geisha's *danna* is a rich, usually married lover. She takes a *danna* only infrequently (though she may have several over her lifetime), traditionally through a special ceremony that resembles a wedding. It is somewhat similar to the ceremony that formalizes the relationship between the Asian Geisha Older Sister and Younger Sister. A geisha would essentially say to all of her clients who tried to go too far with her, "Oh, no, I could only do *that* for my *danna*" (even if she might be less direct in how she communicated the message).

The limitations that you, as an American Geisha, put on the men you are dating (or even on the one Good Man you are engaged to) are similar to the limitations the Asian Geisha puts on her clients. There are certain activities, such as moving in together or some sexual acts, that you may decide to reserve only for your husband. When that is true, you say, "I could only do *that* for my husband."

My married readers probably already have established limits with your husband (or committed Good Man). Think explicitly of what those limits are; write them down. Then, consider whether it might help to revitalize your relationship for you to drop or loosen some of those limitations. I'm not suggesting that you make such changes, only that you *consider* making them.

No Manipulation

The Asian Geisha is not manipulating her clients by reserving certain interactions only for her *danna.* She is not attempting to pressure them into saying, "All right. I'll agree to be your *danna.*" In fact, the most beautiful and accomplished geisha have a good number of clients who would willingly become their *danna,* if only the geisha would allow it. Rather, the Asian Geisha sets limits on her clients for two reasons. First, she has very high standards that must be met by a man who would hope to become her *danna*. Second, and this is a "marketing" consideration, she knows that she must maintain a high-class, selective image in order to continue to attract the best clients, from whom she might eventually choose her *danna*.

As an American Geisha, you, dear Younger Sister, share both of the Asian Geisha's reasons for setting limits on the men you date. Like the Asian Geisha, you have high standards that must be met by any man before you will choose to engage in certain interactions with him. Second, you are aware of maintaining your reputation as classy and selective so you will continue to attract appropriate Good Men. Neither of these reasons for setting limits is meant to manipulate men, my American Geisha trainee; they are meant to assist you in finding the one Good Man whom you chose to be with and who will choose to commit totally to you in marriage.

The Progression of Commitment

As a suitable, rich, older client commits to increasing his financial support for her, the Asian Geisha may be willing to allow him to become her *danna*, to give him her sexual favors on an exclusive basis. You, the American Geisha, are much more generous to your men than the Asian Geisha is. You, Younger Sister, may decide that a Good Man could be any particular age, rich or poor, any class, any race, have any job or any amount of schooling. However, you and your Asian Geisha sister are united in your insistence upon a greater and greater commitment from a man before you become more sexually and emotionally involved with him. Your progression is from a Wrong Man (no commitment and no sex) to a Good Man (monogamous commitment and good sex) to a fiancé (greater commitment and great sex) to a husband (total commitment and outrageous sex). You will, my honest, nonmanipulative Younger Sister, communicate, as appropriate, your own version of how these four relationship stages work for you, so that the men you are involved with know you and your standards, both sexual and other, and can decide whether you inspire them to live up to those standards by committing to you.

The hot, sexy American Geisha knows that when she finds her Good Man, he will be inspired by her unique wonderfulness as an American

Geisha and a Good Woman to make the necessary commitment. Ultimately the right Good Man will love many things about you and will tell you so. "I love how nice you are." "I love your femininity." "I love your vagina." "I love how beautiful you are." Finally, "I love you totally." Or, "I love everything about you."

Learn to say, "I could only do that for my husband" (or "for my fiancé," depending on the stage of your relationship). A quick example: After several months of dating and monogamous sex, your Good Man asks you to move in with him. If you wanted marriage with this Good Man, you might answer, "Oh, I could only do *that* for my husband... or maybe my fiancé." In terms of sexual behavior, perhaps you reserve for your husband performing oral sex on him or swallowing his cum or allowing him to come on your face or anal sex or mild bondage or S & M or sex in a semipublic location or, perhaps, sex while using light recreational drugs ("Oh, I could only trust my *husband* to do that").

Think back to the chapter on female ejaculation. "Shooting" might be your most profoundly intimate and trusting—your most passionate—expression of your sexuality and love. To your Older Sister it seems only quite reasonable that you would choose to reserve sharing that experience with a husband or (it's your choice, of course) with a man you are engaged to.

Here's another scenario to be careful about: Your Good Man asks you to become his fiancé, but he doesn't yet want to get the ring or set the wedding date. You sweetly tell him, "Oh, I could only get engaged if I had a ring and a date for the wedding. That's what an engagement *is,* sweetheart."

Pregnancy and Motherhood

Historically, the Asian Geisha either engaged in unprotected sex or used crude methods of contraception with her *danna,* who usually had his own family. When the geisha became pregnant, she most often had an abortion, sometimes several over the course of a long-term relationship with her *danna.* Sometimes, though, she did carry the child to term. Once the child was born, different arrangements could be made, according to the wishes of the *danna.* Sometimes the child was raised within the *danna*'s family, other times by the geisha with the *danna*'s continuing support. Or she might lose the support of her *danna* and raise the child alone, often while continuing to work as a geisha.

Occasionally a geisha might become pregnant from a personal lover, though having a romantic lover was frowned upon in the Asian Geisha world, especially if he came from a lower socioeconomic class than the men who frequented the geisha-district teahouses. Some unfortunate apprentice geisha became pregnant during their *mizuage,* the ritual taking of their virginity at age thirteen or fourteen by the highest bidder. (This practice was outlawed in Japan in 1958.) It was neither uncommon nor a serious social impropriety for an Asian Geisha to raise a child alone, sometimes more than one. Today, with fewer geisha, the changing roles of women and family in Japan, fewer outrageously wealthy *danna,* and, of course, readily available contraception, accidental pregnancies among geisha are less common.

As an American Geisha, you will probably seek motherhood only within the bond of marriage (and certainly some of you do not seek motherhood at all). Thus, at least until after you are married, dear Younger Sister, you must be sure that you are protected from pregnancy by either your own precautions or the precautions undertaken by the man (assuming you can trust him fully). And if he would choose, perhaps in the heat of passion, to run the risk "just this once" of engaging in sex without contraception, you must tell him firmly, "I could *only* take the risk of getting pregnant with my husband." Again, this limit you put on the relationship is not to manipulate him into marrying you, but to inform him of the standard you have for engaging in sex that could result in pregnancy. To go through the significant physical, emotional, social, and financial changes of a pregnancy requires that you maintain this standard: no pregnancy before marriage. If the man whom you are dating or to whom you are engaged cannot appreciate and totally support your position, then I suggest to you, dear Younger Sister, that he is, at that moment, irresponsible and not a Good Man for you. If, after much discussion and explanation of your position, he still fails to support you enthusiastically, this does not bode well for the future of your relationship or the future of your marriage. If he does not treat your reasonable position with both respect and enthusiasm, I suggest you stop dating him or break the engagement. "I could *only* get pregnant with my husband." Find a Good Man whose enthusiastic response is, "Of course."

Sexually Transmitted Diseases: Absolute Caution!

Whereas the Asian Geisha's business can survive motherhood, she has a more difficult time if she contracts a venereal disease and her clients find out. Rumor of a sexually transmitted disease can lead to a decline in requests for her services.

These days, with the prevalence of AIDS, genital herpes, hepatitis A, B, and C, and HPV (human papillomavirus), it is essential to be very cautious about whom you have sex with. It is one thing for a condom to break and for you to get pregnant. It's another thing for a condom to break and for you to get infected with HIV (human immunodeficiency virus, the AIDS virus), or with HPV (which can cause cervical cancer), or with the hepatitis virus (which attacks the liver and can lead to cancer). Condoms don't fully protect against HSV (herpes simplex virus), which can be located on areas of the body not covered by a condom.

What is a smart and sexy American Geisha to do? Tell your potential Good Man that before you can have sex with him, he must agree to two things: that your relationship will be monogamous, and that before having sex *at all,* both you and he, as a couple, will be medically tested for at least the four STDs I've discussed, and you will share your results with each other. If in fact, Younger Sister, you have chosen a Good Man who truly knows you as the Good Woman you are, then he will understand and respect your caution. He'll also understand that this approach is good for him as well.

If your Good Man has in mind the same long-term goals for the relationship that you do, then postponing sex for two to four weeks and going through the hassle of testing will not be a terribly serious problem for the two of you to deal with. You can still see one another, still kiss, still touch—you just can't be too intimate with his cock or he with your vagina. On the other hand, if, after discussion and explanation, the testing and the waiting seem like unreasonable demands to him, then he is, again, irresponsible and disrespectful of you, and not a Good Man for you. Stop dating him. You say: "I could *only* have sex with a man after we both got checked out." The Good Man says, "I agree. Let's do it."

Five Relationship Stages

Your Older Sister will not attempt to address scenarios for all of the times when you might say something like "I could only do that for my husband." This sentence represents your own high standards and level of self-respect; use it based on your judgment of what is appropriate for you and when. However, it is helpful to spend a little time in forethought so that you can be prepared if you find yourself in certain situations. Below I list five stages of relationships and some phrases that might be useful at each stage.

Situation 1. Dating, before you're sexual with him and before you know if he's a Good Man for you:

"I could only do that (e.g., have sex, pet, meet his parents, go away for the weekend) if we...

...were closer."

...were more committed."

...were seeing only each other."

...decide to keep seeing each other."

...knew each other longer and better."

Situation 2. Dating, before being sexual but after you've determined that he's a Good Man:

"I could only have sex if we agreed to be monogamous and both get tested."

"I could only be sexual with you if I thought we might get married someday."

Situation 3. Dating a Good Man with whom you are sexual:

"I could only do that (e.g., vacation together for two weeks, meet his parents, move in together) if we...

...were engaged."

...knew each other longer."

...were married."

...were more intimate, closer."

...were more committed."

…knew what our future together is."

…were both in love."

Situation 4. You're engaged:

"I could only do that…

…after we were married."

…if I were feeling totally secure about our relationship."

…when I feel totally intimate with you."

Situation 5. You're married:

Even with your husband there may be some limits as to what you are willing to do. Discuss ahead of time, while you are dating and engaged, what your limitations might be. If you are already married, perhaps some of your prohibitions could be relaxed. It's your choice. (Of course, I would never recommend that you agree to the last three on this list!)

"I could never…

…have a sexual threesome."

…do drugs."

…have anal sex."

…let you come in my mouth."

…swallow your cum."

…do bondage (S & M)."

…stop masturbating."

…give up my vibrator."

…stop having 'shooting' orgasms."

Let me close this chapter by returning to the analogy of the cow from Chapter 1. When you and your Good Man are dating, you give him enjoyable, milky sex. When his commitment includes the ring and a wedding date, you offer him wet, creamy sex. After his final commitment of marriage, you enthusiastically smear hot, buttery sex and love all over him. Then your Good Man will experience all that it means for his wife to be a beautiful, hot, sexy, feminine American Geisha.

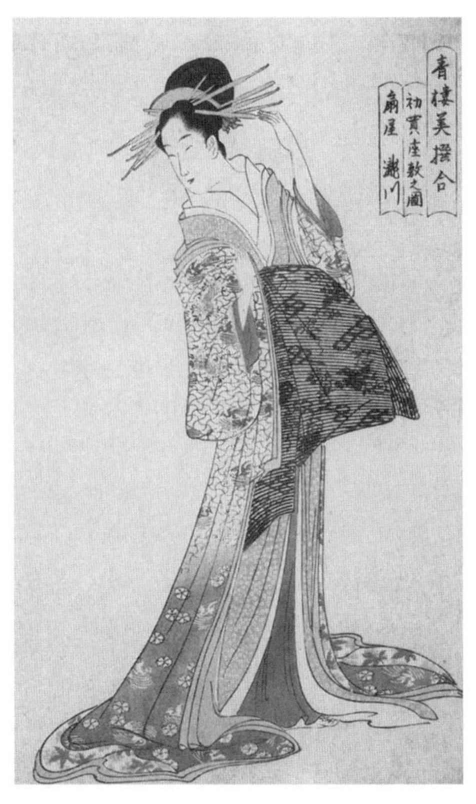

CHAPTER 12

Love Is More than Just Good Sex

Now, Younger Sister, as you are nearing the end of this book and of your training with me, I wish to declare you an Apprentice American Geisha. In Japan, you would be known as a *maiko,* and your Older Sister, feeling that you were ready to go out into the world, would introduce you to many people at parties, meetings, and teahouses. You would be very active, attending events every night.

I cannot do that for you. I cannot be with you. You will introduce yourself alone, of course. And you won't be going to several functions every night. But perhaps you will attend several functions every week in pursuit of your goal of love and marriage. Since I cannot be with you to remind you of your training or to help and guide you when unforeseen circumstances arise, as an Older Sister Asian Geisha would, I want to offer some thoughts that you should keep with you on your way to finding your Good Man, falling in love, and marrying.

Have a Happy, Fun Time while Seeking Love and Marriage

First, always remember that this is a happy and wonderful time for you. Relax. If in my writing I have focused with laserlike intensity on reaching your goals within twelve to eighteen months, don't you focus on that. Instead, focus on enjoying yourself, meeting people, and staying aware of your definition of a Good Man and Your Four Fundamental Needs. Always remember that you are a Good Woman who desires and deserves a Good Man. Stay in the present; enjoy the company of the man or group you are with. Be a happy, fun, relaxed person to spend time with, a woman whose presence reflects her inner confidence and positive optimism. Be an American Geisha.

You Are *Always* Sexy, Even if You're *Not* Always Sexual

If you focus on anything, focus on love. While in your training I have focused somewhat on sex and on being beautiful, feminine, hot, and sexy, I want to remind you again of a fundamental difference between the Asian

Geisha and the American Geisha. In Japan and Korea the Asian Geisha neither seeks nor even believes in love and marriage. By contrast, you, dear Younger Sister Apprentice American Geisha, probably have as a very high priority finding *both* love and marriage with your Good Man.

Remember, too, that the Asian Geisha, although very beautiful, feminine, classy, hot, and sexy to the men who are her well-to-do clients, does not engage in sex very often with those clients. The Asian Geisha keeps her clients satisfied by entertaining them with song, musical instruments, and dance; by conversing intelligently on many topics; by offering her poetry; by serving them drink and food; and, most of all, simply by enchanting her clients with her beautiful and feminine presence at a party, meeting, or dinner. You, too, although beautiful, feminine, classy, hot, and sexy, will not be sexual with many of the men you attract in the course of your search for your Good Man. Instead, you will be an American Geisha version of the Asian Geisha, attracting and beguiling Good Men with your loveliness, charm, and presence until you find the right man for you, your one Good Man to marry. The fortunate few Good Men with whom you choose to engage in a sexual relationship will find an incredible Good Woman who becomes even more sexually responsive and open as her Good Man commits more of himself to her.

I hope the animal sex you choose to have with your Good Man is hot, lusty, frequent, and leads you both to intense, loud, sweaty, fantastic orgasms. However, a really good fuck, or even 365 really good fucks, do not alone create a good, lifelong love relationship and marriage. (It sure can *help* to create that wonderful, happy marriage!)

For my married Apprentice American Geisha, you almost certainly already know from your own experiences that love is a great deal more than just good sex. Keep in mind that we American Geisha need to stay conscious of all the ways we can strengthen our marriages and keep our Good Men attracted to us and satisfied.

Remember the Four Core Characteristics of Your Good Man

First, although your Good Man's values don't have to align perfectly with yours, the fundamental value of honesty and integrity (with you and with others) should be a basic part of his psychological makeup.

Second, as a conscious and aware person yourself, you see that real love and long-term happiness are unlikely if your man does not seek to understand the reality of any situation and then deal responsibly with it.

Third, if this book and my suggestions appeal to you enough for you to have read this far, then you must be a nice woman. There is nothing worse for a nice woman than to be treated unkindly by the man she loves and treats so well. Nice men are nice to everyone because they are nice people. Your evaluation of how nice or not nice a man is will weigh heavily in your judgment of whether he is a Good Man for you.

Finally, make sure the men you date, especially those you choose to sleep with and the one you choose to marry, are happy people, because a marriage to an unhappy (or depressed) man will be an unhappy marriage, guaranteed.

Remember Your Four Fundamental Needs

You must remember that any man will be appropriate for you *only* if he is willing and able to help you fulfill Your Four Fundamental Needs: for marriage and children (if applicable); for mutual love; for sexual passion; and all of this only with a Good Man, of course. If he does want marriage and children, if the two of you are mutually in love, and if there is a hot sexual chemistry between you, then this Good Man is a *very* strong candidate for walking down the aisle, saying "I do," and becoming your husband!

Speak Up for Your Need to Be Married

As you move toward the agreement that the two of you want marriage (and children, if that is true for you), remember that you do not pressure or manipulate your Good Man into marrying you. Instead, as described in Chapter 10, you honestly, fairly, and confidently assert and speak up for what you reasonably need in your life (marriage, kids, love, sex) as a strong, happy, American Geisha woman.

Remember *Your* Characteristics as a Good Woman

Another reminder is about *you*. As you look for that right Good Man to marry, keep part of your focus inward. Stay conscious of yourself as a Good Woman. I've emphasized at some length the qualities you should look for in a Good Man while dealing more in summary with what makes you a Good Woman. Let your Good Man quickly sense that he is in the presence of an honest, conscious, nice, and happy woman. He'll find this Good Woman reflected in the way that you pursue love and marriage. You are honest and conscious about your life goals. You totally refrain from manipulating him, in all phases of your relationship. He can count on dealing with a happy, positive, optimistic person, a woman of good intentions who will always do her best to treat him kindly, fairly, and well. This is a worthy woman. This is a desirable woman, a woman to be pursued, a woman he may want to marry and have bear his children, a Good Woman.

Avoid Aggressive Confrontation

The Asian Geisha tries very hard to avoid confrontation with her clients because of the bad feelings it can bring about and the negative effect it can have on her business relationships long into the future. She does her best to agree to the wishes of her client, unless the request is unreasonable. She is neither frustrated nor resentful that she cannot have her way. Rather, she understands that the nature of her relationship to the client means that she will make all reasonable attempts to comply with his wishes. The Asian Geisha's role is to please and flatter her clients, and to do so both happily and enthusiastically.

Of course, your role in marriage is different. You may want to please and flatter your husband, but he, as a Good Man, should also want to please and flatter you. For your part—and perhaps you could teach him this—always remember that you want to have a positive effect on your relationship. Aggressive confrontation is never sexy; it is more yang than yin. It never brings the two of you closer together. Remember that part of your Geisha Femininity involves being a receptive, nurturing, peaceful woman, even in the middle of any necessary confrontation.

The feminist part of you that gives you backbone cannot always avoid confrontation, even in a great relationship with your Good Man. When it feels right to confront, follow the way of the Asian Geisha and do so *calmly*. Do not confront impulsively. Instead, plan the time and place so as to encourage a calm atmosphere. The Asian Geisha often deals with inebriated clients (little tea and much beer, sake, and whiskey get poured in the teahouses), and is famous for her absolute calm in the midst of chaos or inappropriate, alcohol-fueled behavior on the part of her clients.

Much as the Asian Geisha seeks a gentle resolution that avoids making her client look bad or wrong for his actions or words, your Geisha Calm, coupled with your determination to resolve the situation while allowing your Good Man to save face, can keep a confrontation from becoming an argument. In fact, your Geisha Calm can turn what would otherwise be a confrontation or argument into a *discussion*, which is actually quite yin (oh how we women love to discuss) and even sexy once you reach some agreement.

As a strong American Geisha you must assertively stand up for your most important beliefs. When I ask you to avoid confrontation, I mean that you should not *aggressively* defend your position (nor should your Good Man). Always treat each other with respect and care, and try (both of you) to come from the place of *trusting each other's good intentions*, no matter how entrenched the disagreement might seem to be. Try to follow your Older Sister's ways:

- Do not raise your voice; speak calmly. If his voice gets too loud, ask him gently if he could please speak more softly.
- Keep your face calm, your hands relaxed.
- Seek to have a discussion, not an argument. If he gets more argumentative, always seek to return to a calm discussion.
- Be ready to say you are sorry for how upset both of you are. Often, with your lead giving him permission, a Good Man will express similar feelings.
- Be ready to apologize explicitly for your share of any blame, if doing so can help you get beyond confrontation to working together on the situation.

- Very importantly, remember that an angry, emotional word spoken and heard can never be unspoken and unheard; it lasts in his memory for your entire relationship. Speak very carefully when you are upset. Ask him to do the same.
- Allow your Good Man to save face by nonjudgmentally seeking a solution, not by seeking to place blame on him (even if blaming him seems appropriate and fair).
- Try always to make each other happy, not wrong.
- Ask your Good Man to read this section; then jointly seek to have calm discussions whenever you disagree.

Many books and courses are available that can help you develop skills for dealing with conflict assertively and compassionately in your intimate relationship. When each of you treats the other well, you have the base upon which a great relationship and marriage can be built. All that is required is the somewhat undefinable magic "spark" that leads to emotional love and attraction, and another one that leads to physical chemistry and attraction.

When those two sparks ignite between a Good Man and a Good Woman, can marriage be far away? Assuming your needs are met in his complementary needs, the answer is, "No, marriage cannot be far away." So, let's end this chapter by going back to the sex that is only a *part* of love (yet a very important part). When the engagement ring is on your finger and the wedding date is set (or after the marriage), celebrate the totality of your mutual love by pounding the mattress and shaking the walls with the hottest animal-emotional sex your combined desires can produce.

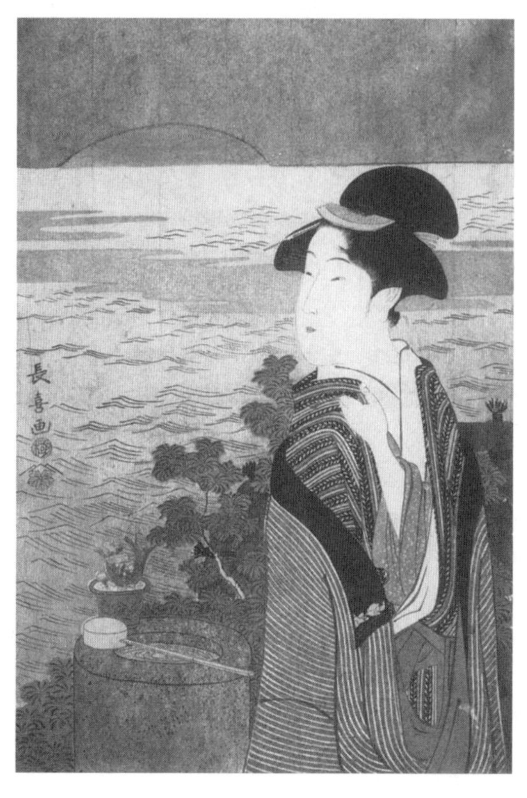

CHAPTER 13

Make the Happiness of Your Marriage Your Highest Priority

When you marry, your journey is not over, is it, sweet Younger Sister? You realize, don't you, without my telling you, that after the wedding ceremony the pleasurable journey continues. If you've spent twelve to eighteen months on the journey to *finding* love and marriage, now your years-long journey will involve *maintaining* a happy, sexy, enthusiastic marriage. Remember that your goal is not to have a great wedding. It is to have a great marriage.

Here, too, there are lessons to be learned from your Asian Sisters. When a gentleman or a company initiates a relationship with a particular teahouse *(ochaya)* or geisha, the relationship often becomes a long-term one, even if sex is never a factor. Many clients that employ the services of the geisha district return again and again to the same teahouse for their functions or request the presence of the same geisha. The relationships sometimes extend to the next generation; clients introduce their sons to their favorite teahouses or geisha, and the sons eventually form their own relationships.

Over time, both the geisha and the women who run the teahouses learn how to make their clients totally satisfied with the services they receive. They get to know the types of dance the men enjoy, the musical instruments they prefer, the sorts of entertainment they wish to see, the games they like to play, the food and caterers they prefer, the brands of alcohol each guest likes, the type of conversation the gentlemen find stimulating, and the level of involvement with the geisha the client expects. They cater to the client's preferred seating arrangements, show the appropriate deference to company VIPs, and determine what mix of *maiko* and senior geisha the client enjoys. With such good care taken of the client's needs and desires, why would he wish to start all over again with another teahouse and a new geisha?

Your Good Man's Greatest Fear: That You'll Change

For centuries, in what is probably one of the earliest examples of "relationship marketing" strategies, teahouse owners and geisha have cultivated these years-long relationships with their clients. This is good business. Clients enjoy the continuity provided by familiar interactions with the geisha.

Likewise, your Good Man hopes that you will remain the loving, beautiful, feminine, kind, sexy American Geisha that you were when he decided, with your subtle help, that he wanted to marry you. Do not disappoint him, dear Younger Sister. Continue forever to be his incredible Good Woman. If you could dig deep into a man's subconscious, you would find that the new groom's greatest fear is that *after the wedding his wife will change.*

Far from completing their training when they become *maiko* or even full geisha, Asian Geisha may continue taking classes for their entire careers. They may learn new entertainment talents, refresh old skills, improve their conversational skills, or educate themselves about subjects that allow them to converse knowledgeably and intelligently with the rich and powerful men who are their clients. (Even Prince Charles, of the British royal family, has been entertained by Japanese geisha.)

Yet, as much as they continue to grow as geisha, they never forget that their primary function is to have that certain presence their clients count on. Though individual geisha change over time, of course, the role of the Asian Geisha has changed little over hundreds of years. The culture of the geisha is known as "the flower and willow world" (*karyukai* in Japanese, a poetic term for the society within the geisha district). The geisha is expected to be as beautiful as a flower and as flexible as a willow, a lovely creature who is aesthetically pleasing to her client's eyes and willing to bend to his particular (but reasonable) wishes. Should the men who patronize the geisha districts have wanted things to change much over the centuries, to become "modernized," the Asian Geisha would probably see it as her duty to accommodate those wishes. This has not happened. Clients desire that the geisha *not* change; they want her to continue to represent the traditional ways.

Make Your Good Man Feel Lucky That He Married You

Do you sense where I am leading you, dear Younger Sister? Your Good Man married his American Geisha because of all you brought to him that gave him such pleasure: your sweetness, your niceness, your love, your beauty, your femininity, your sexiness, your sexuality. Now that you are married, he wants to continue to experience all of these pleasures. As the Asian Geisha focuses on continuing to please even her longtime clients, so should you focus on continuing to please your husband even after you are married. Your beauty, femininity, and sexuality are very important parts of your marriage. Take care of yourself, your husband, and your marriage. You were excited about *getting* married. Now stay excited about *being* married.

You have attracted and married your Good Man, the best man for you. You are so happy. You are so lucky. You *made* your own luck. But you feel fortunate to have found and married such a great Good Man. He, too, no doubt is happy to be married to such a great Good Woman. He's a lucky man. You want him always to feel fortunate that he found and married you. You want to continue to treat him so wonderfully that he frequently says to you, "I'm so lucky I married you."

If you are already married, I hope your wonderful husband *does* tell you over and over how happy and lucky he is to be married to you. If you, dear married American Geisha, have read this far in a book where you are a secondary audience to my primary audience of single women, I know that you are incredibly motivated to have a fantastic relationship with your husband. He *is* lucky to have you as his wife. Just as the willow bends and changes yet remains a willow, I only suggest that you imagine ways to bend and change that will allow you to remain the fabulous woman he married ten months or ten years (or fifty years!) ago. All the while, keep the knowledge in your heart that he is lucky that he married you!

In the midst of all of this happiness and celebration, Younger Sister Apprentice American Geisha, please listen to your Older Sister for just a few more words of advice about your marriage. You and I both know what happens to more than half of American marriages: They end in divorce, which means they end with love lost, beauty only a memory, femininity abandoned, kindheartedness turned to anger, sexuality long departed. And many more couples do not divorce but live out diminished or loveless lives together, perhaps an even worse fate. There must be a hundred or a thousand or a million different reasons for those marriages to have failed. I want you as an American Geisha to avoid this painful unhappiness, of course.

The goal of this book is not just to help you get married, but to help you keep your husband happy and help you to be a happy wife, forever. Once again, hearing a little bit of my own story may be helpful.

My Failure as a Sweet, Sexy Wife for My Husband

After Rich and I married, in April 2000, we began to plan for a baby. Rich, who is twenty years older than I, had never been married and had no children. Our desire to have children meant he had to have a twenty-five-year-old vasectomy reversed. Well, Rich was a little slow to schedule his scrotum to go under the surgeon's knife (perhaps understandably!). But he did do it. By August 2003 we were informally paying attention to my fertility cycles, then happily fucking like bunnies to give ourselves the best chances of getting pregnant. By December 2004 we were still not pregnant. We decided to try in vitro fertilization. We chose to work with a well-respected Korean fertility clinic in Los Angeles. Unfortunately, Rich's sperm were mostly "floaters," not "swimmers," and my egg-retrieval procedure, a lengthy, painful process involving multiple needle shots into my stomach and butt, produced only one egg, which did not mature and therefore could not be mixed "in vitro" (in a petri dish) with Rich's underperforming sperm. The doctor's opinion was that an attempt at a second lengthy, painful, and expensive egg-retrieval procedure would probably fail to produce more or better eggs.

We decided to forego any further attempts to have our own child, and we decided not to adopt. Rich probably embraced the "no kids" mindset better and faster than I did. I grew clinically depressed for a while. What could I do since I would not have a child to raise for the next eighteen years? How could I fill the void of unfulfilled expectations? My life felt empty.

An idea developed in me. If I couldn't give birth to a baby, I would fill the void by "giving birth to" a book about the Asian secrets I had learned. I thought they would be as helpful to other women who were pursuing love and marriage as they had proven to be to me. Rich thought the book was a good idea.

So far, so good. Now, here is the cautionary part of my tale.

I became obsessed with the book (*this* book). I stayed up almost every night until 3:00, 4:00, or 5:00 A.M., leaving Rich to go to bed alone hours earlier. I would get up at 10:00 A.M. for my part-time middle-school teaching job. Rich tried to be supportive at first. But my total focus on writing continued. Nothing else mattered. If I couldn't be a mom, I was determined to be a published author.

Rich encouraged me to come to bed with him and to get up early to do my research and writing. Somehow this didn't work for me. With my energy focused only on writing, writing, writing, I just wasn't tired at a normal bedtime.

Rich expressed some upset and disappointment, but I hardly noticed. Our very active sex life fell to pieces. Going out together became infrequent because I wanted to write. This probably went on for five or six months, until one night my hurt and angry husband told me that he felt abandoned. "We are like roommates now, not lovers, not husband and wife," Rich complained. He told me he missed the woman he had married five years ago.

"I guess I've changed. People do change, you know," I responded distractedly.

"I miss the woman I married," he repeated. "I miss the woman I love, the woman whose highest priority was our relationship."

"I can't be the same person now that I know I am infertile," I said, choking on my words.

"Your writing is ruining our marriage. You care about your damned book more than you care about our marriage."

I couldn't understand why he thought that our marriage had gotten in trouble because of my passion for writing. I shot back that he didn't support me and my writing.

"Your book is about how to make a man and a husband happy. But as the author, you need to know that your own marriage is in danger."

I stood there, stunned. What's the point of writing a relationship book when my own man is not happy and my own marriage is in danger?

For the last few months, I hadn't been able to bear the thought that I had failed as a woman. I was haunted by the idea that "you can't be fully a woman until you become a mother." Now my husband was telling me that I had also failed as a wife.

I asked Rich for help. I realized that I wanted to get away from my all-consuming preoccupation with writing. I needed a husband, not just a roommate. He needed me back as his wife, a woman at least somewhat similar to the one he had married five years earlier. He wanted a nice, sweet, sexy wife, not an obsessed writer.

I saw that I had gotten involved in a rebound love affair after I found out that I couldn't get pregnant. At least that's how Rich interpreted my consuming passion to write a book—as an affair that caused me to "cheat" on him and give my attention to another love. Writing a book was replacing the real love affair I had with my husband. As he listened, Rich for the first time understood how hard I had taken the loss of my goal of motherhood.

In the end, Rich agreed enthusiastically to support my writing, even acting as my first-draft editor, and I happily committed to refocusing on our marriage as my highest priority while still pursuing my writing.

It's still not easy to accept that at age forty-three I will never be a mother. But out of this experience I gained both a recharged marriage and an ongoing passion for writing.

Your Husband and Your Relationship as Your Highest Priority

Oh, dear Younger Sister, I was such a fool to have forgotten what Rich and I had agreed to even before we got married (and which we had put in writing and had read to one another as part of our wedding vows): that the strength and happiness of our marriage would be our very highest priority, always.

I had forgotten what brought me my greatest happiness: my wonderful relationship with my Good Man husband. My strongest advice for you after your marriage, dear Younger Sister, is to keep the quality of your love relationship with your husband as your highest priority. Very importantly, share this chapter with your Good Man well before your marriage. Encourage him to make the same commitment to you. As a couple, promise to remain conscious of the quality of your relationship as the most important thing to you, individually and together.

It is too easy to allow the quality of your marriage to slip to a lower priority. Careers, friends, in-laws, children, and hobbies will all tug at your kimono sleeve to demand your time and attention. This is life. It is full of things other than your relationship that can command your focus. As an American Geisha, you have a more difficult undertaking than does the Asian Geisha, who can keep her clients as her highest priority because she does not marry or plan a family. You marry and want a family, yet you probably also have a job or even an engaging career that pulls your attention away from your relationship with your Good Man husband. Fight successfully to maintain an active love life. Stay beautiful and feminine. Always be nice to each other.

Even your children should be a second priority. They should come some distance behind your priority of maintaining a deep, mutual love relationship with your Good Man. Remember, as a psychologist once said, "The very best thing mothers or fathers can do for their children is to be actively, enthusiastically, and mutually in love with their spouses."

Another part of keeping your marriage as your highest priority is to celebrate your anniversary. Make it a memorable day of renewal of your love and commitment to one another. Perhaps return to your honeymoon spot. Review your original wedding vows. Write new, updated vows. Stay excited about your mutual love.

Express Your Love Daily

Every day, kiss and verbally express your love; touch and make love frequently. An American Geisha knows that both men and women need, enjoy, and appreciate frequent reassurance that they are loved and physically desired. You two can never reassure each other of these things too many times. I repeat, dear Younger Sister, it is *never* too often or too soon to say to your spouse:

I love you.

I like who you are.

You make me so happy.

I'm so glad I married you.

I'm so lucky to have married you.

You have a beautiful body.

You're the only one I could ever love.

You get more beautiful every day (him to you).

You are so beautiful (him to you).

You are such a good lover (you to him).

You're so nice (good, sweet) to me.

I love being alone with you.

I'm so glad you are in my life.

You're always so supportive of me.

You're such a good wife (husband).

Rules for Spouses

So that you and your husband stay aware of, involved in, and excited about your marriage, I want to suggest some "rules" for both of you. Review them from time to time and add whatever additional ones you like:

RULES FOR A MARRIED WOMAN

- Be enthusiastically available to your man whenever he wants you sexually.
- Be nice.
- Be sweet.
- Tell him directly what you are thinking. He misses subtle messages.
- Love to softly touch his cock when it's not hard.
- Kiss and suck his cock without his asking. Exercise no restraint. Eat it all!
- Tell your friends positive things about your husband, and believe them.
- Stay beautiful.
- Be assertive about what you need and want, including sexually.
- Be soft and feminine with your husband.
- Make your relationship, not your individual needs, your highest priority.

- Find ways to make him your hero.
- Always respect your man, be he rich or poor, C.E.O. or day laborer.
- Don't try to fix his problems unless he asks for help.
- Don't compare your husband's income, cock, or job title to those of your friends' husbands or of your ex—unless your man's is bigger.
- Have good intentions. When you trust each other's good intentions, there is no anger, even when mistakes are made.
- Learn to be assertive and direct yet kind and noncritical in your communications.
- Don't ask him about his masturbation fantasies, and don't be jealous of them.
- Consider telling him about your masturbation fantasies involving woman's rock-hard nipples (or other lesbian fantasies).
- Let him watch you masturbate.
- Watch him masturbate (and participate a little).

RULES FOR A MARRIED MAN

- Wear your wedding ring 24/7.
- Be nice.
- Do household chores before she asks.
- Let her go out with her girlfriends and occasionally stay overnight with them.
- Let her have a weekend trip with her girlfriends.
- Let her know you cherish and love her.
- Call her at work just to say "I love you."
- Listen to her problems without seeking solutions.
- Phone home if you will be late.
- Send her flowers at work so she can get them in front of her coworkers.
- Send a love letter to her workplace.
- Show your affection by kissing and hugging in front of her friends.

- Tell her often, "You're beautiful," and that you love her.
- Brag to your male friends about your wife; tell her you've done so.
- Make your relationship, not your job or career, your highest priority.
- Don't spend too much time on the newspaper, the TV, or your buddies.
- Buy her perfume that *you* like.
- Place a picture of her (at least one) in your office or work space.

RULES FOR A MARRIED COUPLE

- Never go to bed angry at each other. Forgive.
- Go to bed at the same time.
- Sleep in the same bed.
- Sleep naked, always.
- At least kiss and hug before you sleep, always.
- Always have good intentions toward your spouse in whatever you do. (I know I am repeating this one. It's worth repeating.)
- Do things together.
- Be quiet together, comfortably.
- Feel fortunate and happy you found each other.
- Laugh together.

Always Stay Geisha Beautiful and Feminine As You Age

Once a woman is beautiful and feminine, she never needs to lose those qualities as she ages. We have all seen beautiful, feminine women in their sixties and seventies, even perhaps in their eighties. As an American Geisha you will always make the maintenance of your beauty and femininity a high priority, investing the time and money necessary to do so no matter what your age. Stay aware of this goal, and proud that you want to be at your best as a woman at any age. Some of you may choose to undergo surgery to help you remain beautiful; however, I want you to know that you can quite naturally retain your best American Geisha qualities for your entire life. Men and women will comment on your attractiveness, charm, and kindheartedness, and mourners at your graveside will smile as they recall how you maintained these traits even in the last years of your long, happy life with your Good Man.

Your training is complete, dear Younger Sister. Go forth with confidence and a happy smile.

You are now an American Geisha.

AFTERWORD

"Geisha Power": Find Your Sexuality and Keep Your Good Man

You've finished reading *Sex Secrets of an American Geisha.* I hope you, my dear Younger Sister, found it to be a practical book, not merely theoretical, with ideas that you can really use in seeking and satisfying your Good Man. You have adopted a Geisha Consciousness and have become Geisha Attractive. Along the way, I've asked you to think and to write about your goals and what you want from a Good Man. If you have simply read straight through and haven't taken the quiet time to do that thinking, feeling, and writing, please do it now. This book will help you to be married within twelve-to-eighteen months, but only if you *do* what is suggested, only if you *use* the Asian Geisha's secrets.

I've asked you to buy certain items, the vibrator being the most important, and to become familiar with your vagina, and to masturbate, *now.* If you have not done any (or any one) of these things, please begin, *now.* Again, to marry quickly, you must *act* on these secrets; you must *do* what is required to attract, satisfy, and keep your Good Man.

Once you begin to *act* and to *do,* to *use* these hot, sexy Asian Geisha secrets (all of which are action verbs), you begin to change your Geisha Consciousness, incorporating into it more of that person you are becoming, an American Geisha. Do it now, please. *Today,* begin your journey to sexuality, love, and marriage to your Good Man.

Good luck from your American Geisha Older Sister in your search for your Good Man and in finding the happiness, love, and marriage that you deserve as a Good Woman.

I want to know how I've helped you. Visit my website, at www.AmericanGeishaHouse.com, and share with me your success story of love, sex, and marriage. Tell me what is working for you.

Even invite me to your wedding. I promise I'll at least send you a personal message in return.

GLOSSARY

A Hot and Sexy List of Terms

American Geisha: the author's term for a woman who uses Asian Geisha wisdom and secrets in her pursuit of sexuality, love, and marriage with a Good Man; the author is the first or Older Sister American Geisha, and the reader is invited to become a trainee or Younger Sister American Geisha.

anterior vaginal wall: the front wall of the vagina (the top wall when a woman is lying on her back); where the G-spot is located.

areola: the pink-brown, sometimes rough-to-the-touch ring of flesh surrounding the nipple.

Asian fetish: being particularly attracted to Asian women, often due to the stereotypes concerning them. Also called "yellow fever."

Asian Geisha: author's term for the blending of the Japanese *geisha* and the Korean *kisaeng.*

Asian Geisha's training: learning the art of conversation, dance, song, music (*shamisen* and drums), tea ceremony, dressing, flower arrangement, poetry, walking, entering a room, pouring drinks, serving food, and much more.

blended orgasm: see "G-spot orgasm."

blow job: fellatio; sucking and licking the cock (and balls) to please a man and to bring him to orgasm.

bondage: voluntary tying up of your man before having your sexy way with him; or vice versa.

calories in and out: a fundamental law of physics. If you consume fewer calories in a day than you burn up, you will lose weight that day; and vice versa.

cervix: the neck of the uterus, which connects it to the vagina. Deep cock thrusting can reach the cervix.

clitoral orgasm: the pudendal nerves send messages of sexual arousal from the clitoris to the brain, eventually resulting in a clitoral orgasm, which involves the contraction of the front two-thirds of the PC muscles. Female ejaculation will not accompany strictly clitoral orgasms.

clitoris: one of the centers of sensual/sexual feeling in the woman, located where the inner vulval lips join just below the mound of Venus; covered by the clitoral hood; becomes engorged with blood when sexually excited; involved in both clitoral and blended orgasms.

coccyx bone: the tailbone, located at the base of the spine and to which one end of the pubococcygeus (PC) muscles attach.

cock: preferred sexual name for the penis ("penis" is a urological term).

conscious relationship: a continued focus on and awareness of the state or quality of your love relationship.

danna: patron, supporter, sponsor; the lover for whom a Japanese geisha saves her greatest commitment of attention, time, and sexuality; the relationship is formalized through a marriagelike ceremony.

erectile dysfunction: when the male has difficulty getting or maintaining a satisfactory erection.

erectile tissue: network of tissue in the genital areas of both men and women that fills with blood or other liquid and swells when either indirectly or directly stimulated during sexual arousal; includes the urethral sponge in women.

female ejaculation: emission through the urethra of a nonurine fluid stored in the urethral sponge during indirect arousal of the female prostate through direct stimulation of the G-spot (in this book the ejaculate is also called Gräfenberg Juice, Love Juice, Feminine Waters, Love Lava, Feminine Fountain).

female prostate: formerly known as the Skene's glands, a network of glands and ducts surrounding the urethra and bladder. The engorgement of the female prostate with blood can be felt from within the vagina by applying direct pressure against the area of the upper vaginal wall known as the G-spot.

female prostate orgasm: see "G-spot orgasm."

female sexual anatomy (organs): includes the clitoris, urethra, vagina, vulva, prostate, G-spot, pelvic muscles and nerves, and other erectile tissues.

feminine-ist: a woman who happily operates out of her sense of her femininity; not to be confused with *feminist,* which is practically the opposite of feminine-ist.

flower and willow world: the Asian Geisha life; geisha society; the geisha district; the geisha world; poetically, *karyukai* in Japanese.

Four Core Characteristics of a Good Man: four traits a Good Man has as a basic part of his personality; nonnegotiable characteristics you seek in a Good Man: 1) has good values; 2) is aware and responsible; 3) is nice and treats you well; and 4) is a happy person.

Four Fundamental Needs, Your: absolute, basic needs in your relationship with your Good Man: 1) need to marry; 2) need for a strong love relationship; 3) need for a passionate sexual relationship; and 4) need for only a Good Man to date and marry.

geisha: Japanese artist entertainer; in Korea, *kisaeng.*

Geisha Attitude: particular attitude toward men, similar to the attitude of the Japanese geisha toward her male clients. See "Geisha Consciousness."

Geisha Attractiveness: the combination of an Asian Geisha's or American Geisha's physical beauty, beautiful clothes, sexiness, and femininity.

Geisha Consciousness: developing a way of thinking like an Asian Geisha, particularly toward men; understanding geisha ways of looking at the male-female relationship.

Geisha Femininity: an appreciation that the Asian Geisha has the power of her femininity in relationship with men; the Asian Geisha is seen as the embodiment of femininity (which the American Geisha also seeks).

Geisha Plan: American Geisha Weight Loss and Maintenance Plan; not a diet.

Good Man: Mr. Right, Prince Charming, a near-perfect-for-you man, an appropriate man for your future husband. He has the Four Core Characteristics; the only type of man to date or marry. See "Four Core Characteristics of a Good Man."

Good Woman: You, the reader, the American Geisha; has the same Four Core Characteristics as the Good Man; a woman worthy of finding a Good Man; the type of woman sought by Good Men.

Gräfenberg Juice: after the doctor who first clinically identified the G-spot, the juice or liquid that is ejaculated following G-spot stimulation; Love Juice, Feminine Waters, Love Lava, Feminine Fountain.

G-spot: small, slightly raised, sexually sensitive area located one and a half to two inches inside the vagina on the front wall; associated with the female prostate and female ejaculation. Clinically identified in the 1950s by German physician Ernst Gräfenberg.

G-spot orgasm: the physical and emotional sensations and climax created by simultaneous stimulation of the clitoris and the G-spot; often involves female ejaculation; also known as a blended orgasm.

female prostate orgasm: same as G-spot orgasm.

inner and outer vulval lips: labia minora and labia majora, respectively.

Kegel exercises: a set of biofeedback exercises originally designed by Dr. Arnold Kegel to strengthen the pubococcygeus (PC) muscles to reduce urinary stress incontinence; they also strengthen the grip of the vagina; strength of these muscles is critical to the ability to female ejaculate.

kisaeng: in Korea, the equivalent of the Japanese geisha.

labia majora: outer vulval lips; defines the outer limits of the vaginal area, like a raised curb; swells some with sexual stimulation.

labia minora: inner "butterflylike" vulval lips, composed of thin, very sensitive skin that often swells and engorges quite noticeably with sexual stimulation; lie inside the labia majora.

latent sexuality: becoming aware of one's sexual potential later in life.

Lucky Seven development areas: to be 1) positive, optimistic, and happy; 2) relaxed, at ease, confident (not desperate); 3) sexually aware of your desires and capabilities; 4) at just the right weight; 5) fit, toned, healthy; 6) beautiful and feminine; and 7) dressed and made up well.

maiko: in Japan, younger sister; geisha-in-training; apprentice geisha.

manhood: cock; also, a man's psychological identity tied to his cock.

masturbate/masturbation: playing with yourself; stimulation of your own genitals to achieve orgasm. Sometimes involves using sex toys; sometimes in front of your partner.

mizuage: in Japan, the ritual taking of a *maiko*'s virginity by the highest bidder (now illegal).

monogamous: having a committed relationship with only one sex partner.

mound of Venus: the fleshy mound over the pubic bone above the clitoris, often covered in pubic hair.

obi: wide, heavy sash worn with a kimono.

ochaya: teahouse, where the *maiko* and geisha often entertain clients. More sake and scotch are served than tea.

okiya: geisha house, where the geisha family (geisha, "mother," cook, maids, and *maiko*) lives.

Older Sister: the author's role in this book; trains the apprentice geisha *(maiko)*.

onesan: older sister in a geisha family; guides and trains a *maiko.*

orgasm: a climax reached during sexual excitement; coming. The peak of sexual excitement usually accompanied by muscle contractions and ejaculation in the male, or by muscle contractions and possible ejaculation in the female.

pelvic nerve: connects to the bladder, uterus, urethra, female prostate, and the lower spinal cord; involved in the more rare and very emotional uterine orgasm, usually with no female ejaculation; also involved in G-spot orgasm.

prostate gland: in the male, the gland that surrounds the neck of the bladder and the urethra, and which produces seminal fluid. In the female, the organ that is felt through the vaginal wall when pressing on the G-spot inside the vagina; also involved in producing the larger quantity of female ejaculate.

pubococcygeus muscles (PC muscles): "love muscles," vaginal muscles; a set of pelvic muscles in both the man and the woman that aid ejaculation and cause the contractions in an orgasm; also control the urinary steam. They run from the pubic bone to the coccyx bone (tailbone) and help to support the pelvic floor. Contraction of these muscles makes possible female ejaculation and G-spot orgasm.

pudendal nerve: responds to stimulation around the clitoris, labia, and vaginal entrance, as well as the front portion of the PC muscles; involved in clitoral and G-spot orgasms.

quiet place: place of contemplation to become aware of your deepest and most fundamental needs and desires in a relationship with a man.

reservoir of ejaculate liquid: in women the urethral sponge, located near the female prostate.

seminal fluid: the fluid from the male prostate that mixes with sperm and is ejaculated from the cock during orgasm; a somewhat similar fluid may be ejaculated by the woman after G-spot stimulation.

sense of class: attention to the classy image you always want to convey with your combination of beauty (you plus your clothes), femininity, and sexiness.

sexual animal: you and all animals are physical and sexual creatures; a reminder to enjoy our bodies and to enjoy sex as freely and totally as the lower animals do, without inhibition.

sex toys: sex aid; any object used to bring about or enhance sexual arousal or orgasm. The basic sex toy is the vibrator.

shooting: also called squirting, gushing, flooding, emitting. Explosive, volcanic release of Gräfenberg Juice; the female ejaculation.

shrine: small bedroom area devoted to worshiping your Good Man's cock.

Skene's glands: named after Dr. Alexander Skene; a small group of glands and ducts surrounding the urethra; now acknowledged as the female prostate; involved in female ejaculation.

Taoism: (pronounced "dow-ism") A Chinese religion and philosophy based on the teachings of Lao-tse (sixth century B.C.), that advocates simplicity and selflessness.

testicles: balls, testes. The two male sex glands located in the scrotum.

urethra: urethral canal; urinary tract. The canal or tube that carries urine from the bladder; also serves as the passageway for the ejection of ejaculate in both males and females. In women it runs from the bladder to the urethral opening; in men it runs from the bladder to the tip of the penis.

urethral opening: where urine and ejaculate exit the body; in women, located between the clitoris and the vaginal opening.

urethral sponge: See "erectile tissue."

uterine muscles: a section of the PC muscles that lies close to the coccyx; involved in the rare uterine orgasm.

uterine orgasm: reached through stimulation of the pelvic nerve and depends upon deep, strong cock thrusting that jostles the cervix and indirectly stimulates the uterine muscles. This orgasm seems to have the most intense emotional component. It is much less likely to involve female ejaculation.

uterus: womb; contains the developing fetus; involved in some orgasms.

vagina: the soft, short passageway that leads from a woman's vulva to her cervix.

vaginal walls: interior portion of the vagina; secretes lubricating fluid (which makes a woman "wet").

vulva: a woman's external sex organs (clitoris, clitoral hood, labia majora, labia minora).

yang: represents the masculine (from Taoism).

yellow fever: see "Asian fetish."

Yellow Emperor: a legendary Chinese ruler (approximately 2600 B.C.); he figured prominently in the medical and sexological teachings of Taoism nearly 2,000 years later.

Yellow Emperor's female sex expert: Su Nu, the Elemental Maid, one of the most widely quoted instructresses in Taoist sex; she is credited with authoring several sexual handbooks.

yin: represents the feminine (from Taoism).

Younger Sister: the reader's role in learning the American Geisha's secrets from the author; similar to the role of *maiko* (apprentice) in a geisha family.

zodiac: fate and destiny as foretold and unfolded by four pillars: the year, month, day, and time you are born; a way to passively wait for life to happen, surrendering to fate without specific future plans.

Resources and Recommended Readings

Author Contact Information

Website: www.AmericanGeishaHouse.com

E-mail: pykimconant@yahoo.com

Must-Haves

The following resources are particularly recommended:

BOOKS

Downer, Lesley. *Women of the Pleasure Quarters: The Secret History of the Geisha.* New York: Broadway Books, 2002. A Westerner's inside view of the geisha life.

Ladas, Alice K., Beverly Whipple, and John Perry. *The G Spot and Other Discoveries about Human Sexuality.* New York: Owl Books, 2005. Presents the science behind the female prostate and female ejaculation.

Sundahl, Deborah. *Female Ejaculation and the G-Spot.* Alameda, CA: Hunter House, 2003. Excellent book to aid you in becoming a "shooter." See especially pages 45–46 and 93, concerning the rare uterine orgasm.

Venning, Rachel, and Claire Cavanah. *Sex Toys 101: A Playfully Uninhibited Guide.* New York: Fireside, 2003. A large-size book full of colorful illustrations of sex-toy products.

DVD

Dr. Susan Block's *Dr. Suzy's Squirt Salon.* Available through the website www.drsusanblock.com. Extremely frank and truly educational 2½-hour video. Absolutely the best instruction for becoming a female ejaculator.

VIBRATOR

Pocket Rocket, available in most sex and romance shops, as well as online at www.babeland.com, www.adameve.com, and www.thepleasurechest.com.

Recommended Reading

The following books were helpful to me in writing *Sex Secrets of an American Geisha* and may be useful to you as further reading:

RELATIONSHIPS, MARRIAGE, AND SEX

Allen, Patricia, and Sandra Harmon. *Getting to "I Do."* New York: William Morrow, 1994.

Altalida, Lisa. *Dating Boot Camp.* New York: Alpha Books, 2004.

Around, Miriam, and Samuel Pauker. *The First Year of Marriage: What to Expect, What to Accept, and What You Can Change for a Lasting Marriage.* New York: Warner Books, 1996.

Bawden, Jennifer. *Get a Life, Then Get a Man: A Single Woman's Guide.* New York: Plume Books, 2000.

Behrendt, Greg, and Liz Tuccillo. *He's Just Not That Into You.* New York: Simon Spotlight Entertainment, 2004.

Bodansky, Vera, and Steve Bodansky. *Extended Massive Orgasm.* Alameda, CA: Hunter House, 2000.

———. *To Bed or Not to Bed.* Alameda, CA: Hunter House, 2006.

Brothers, Joyce. *What Every Woman Ought to Know about Love and Marriage.* New York: Ballantine Books, 1984.

———. *What Every Woman Should Know about Men.* New York: Ballantine Books, 1992.

Brown, Sandra L. *How to Spot a Dangerous Man Before You Get Involved.* Alameda, CA: Hunter House, 2005.

Buss, David M. *The Evolution of Desire: Strategies of Human Mating.* New York: Basic Books, 1994.

Cox, Tracey. *Hot Sex: How to Do It.* New York: Bantam Books, 1999.

———. *Hot Relationships: How to Know What You Want, Get What You Want, and Keep It Red Hot.* New York: Bantam Books, 2000.

Daily, Lisa. *Stop Getting Dumped.* New York: Plume Books, 2001.

De Angelis, Barbara. *Secrets about Men Every Woman Should Know.* New York: Dell Publishing, 1991.

———. *Are You the One for Me?* New York: Dell Publishing, 1997.

———. *Ask Barbara: The 100 Most-Asked Questions about Love, Sex, and Relationships.* New York: Delacorte Press, 1997.

Fein, Ellen, and Sherrie Schneider. *The Rules for Marriage.* New York: Warner Books, 2001.

Feldhahn, Shaunti. *For Women Only: What You Need to Know about the Inner Lives of Men.* Sisters, OR: Multnomah Publishers, 2004.

Gerstman, Bradley, Christopher Pizzo, and Rich Seldes. *What Men Want.* New York: Quill, 2000.

Goldberg, Herb. *What Men Really Want.* New York: Signet Books, 1991.

Gottman, John M., and Nan Silver. *The Seven Principles for Making Marriage Work.* New York: Three Rivers Press, 1999.

Grant, Toni. *Being a Woman: Fulfilling Your Femininity and Finding Love.* New York: Avon Books, 1989.

Gray, John. *Men Are from Mars, Women Are from Venus.* New York: HarperCollins, 1992.

———. *Men, Women, and Relationships.* New York: HarperCollins, 1993.

———. *Mars and Venus on a Date.* New York: HarperCollins, 1997.

Hendrix, Harville. *Getting the Love You Want: A Guide for Couples.* New York: Harper and Row, 1990.

James, Larry. *How to Really Love the One You're With.* Scottsdale, AZ: Career Assurance Press, 1994.

Keesling, Barbara. *How to Make Love All Night (and Drive a Woman Wild)*. New York: HarperCollins, 1995.

———. *Sexual Pleasure: Reaching New Heights of Sexual Arousal and Intimacy*, 2nd ed. Alameda, CA: Hunter House, 2005.

Kent, Margaret. *How to Marry the Man of Your Choice*. New York: Warner Books, 2005.

Leonardi, Tom. *Secrets of Sensual Lovemaking: The Ultimate in Female Ecstasy*. New York: Signet/Penguin Group, 1995.

Locker, Sari. *The Complete Idiot's Guide to Being Sexy*. Indianapolis, IN: Alpha Books, 2001.

Masterton, Graham. *Drive Him Wild: A Hands-On Guide to Pleasuring Your Man in Bed*. New York: Signet/Penguin Group, 1993

———. *How to Drive Your Man Wild in Bed*. New York: A Signet Book/Penguin Group, 1976.

Moore, Myreah, and Jodie Gould. *Date Like a Man: What Men Know about Dating and Are Afraid You'll Find Out*. New York: Quill, HarperCollins, 2001.

Nakamoto, Steve. *Men Are Like Fish*. Huntington Beach, CA: Java Books, 2002.

Norwood, Robin. *Women Who Love Too Much*. New York: Pocket Books, 1997.

Outcalt, Todd. *Before You Say "I Do": Important Questions for Couples to Ask Before Marriage*. New York: Perigee Books, 1998.

Paget, Lou. *How to Give Her Absolute Pleasure*. New York: Broadway Books, 2000.

Penney, Alexandra. *How to Make Love to a Man*. New York: Dell Books, 1982.

Rabin, Susan. *How to Attract Anyone, Anytime, Anyplace*. New York: Plume/Penguin, 1993.

St. Claire, Olivia. *203 Ways to Drive a Man Wild in Bed*. New York: Harmony Books, 1993.

Schlessinger, Laura. *The Proper Care and Feeding of Husbands*. New York: HarperCollins, 2004.

EASTERN/ASIAN/ORIENTAL SEXOLOGY

Anand, Margo. *The Art of Sexual Ecstasy: The Path of Sacred Sexuality for Western Lovers*. New York: Tarcher/Putnam, 1989.

Bacarr, Jina. *The Japanese Art of Sex: How to Tease, Seduce, and Pleasure the Samurai in Your Bedroom*. Berkeley, CA: Stone Bridge Press, 2004.

Chang, Jolan. *The Tao of Love and Sex: The Ancient Chinese Way to Ecstasy*. New York: Compass/Penguin, 1991.

Chu, Valentin. *The Yin-Yang Butterfly: Ancient Chinese Sexual Secrets for Western Lovers*. New York: Tarcher/Putnam, 1994.

Douglas, Nik, and Penny Slinger. *Sexual Secrets: The Alchemy of Ecstasy*. Rochester, VT: Destiny Books, 1979.

Gach, Michael Reed. *Acupressure for Lovers*. New York: Bantam Books, 1997.

Lai, Hsi. *The Sexual Teachings of the White Tigress: Secrets of the Female Taoist Masters*. Rochester, VT: Destiny Books, 2001.

Levy, Howard S., and Akira Ishihara. *The Tao of Sex*. Lower Lake, CA: Integral Publishing, 1989.

Lightwoman, Leora. *Tantra: The Path to Blissful Sex*. London: Piatkus, 2004.

Prasso, Sheridan. *The Asian Mystique*. New York: Public Affairs, 2005.

Sudo, Philip Toshio. *Zen Sex: The Way of Making Love*. New York: HarperCollins, 2000.

Zettnersan, Chian. *Taoist Bedroom Secrets*. Twin Lakes, WI: Lotus Press, 2002.

THE WORLD OF THE GEISHA

Dalby, Liza. *Geisha*. Berkeley and Los Angeles, CA: University of California Press, 1998.

Geisha Secrets: A Pillow Book for Lovers (Eddison Sadd Editions). New York: Carroll and Graf, 2000.

Golden, Arthur. *Memoirs of a Geisha* (Vintage Contemporaries movie tie-in edition). New York: Vintage, 2005.

Iwasaki, Mineko. *Geisha: A Life*. New York: Atria Books, 2002.

Louis, Lisa. *Butterflies of the Night: Mama-Sans, Geisha, Strippers, and the Japanese Men They Serve*. New York: Tengu Books, 1992.

Index

I

J

K

L

M

N

O

P

R

S

T

U

V

W

Y

More Hunter House Books on SEXUALITY & ORGASM

FEMALE EJACULATION & THE G-SPOT

by Deborah Sundahl ... Forewords by Annie Sprinkle and Alice Ladas

Discover the G-spot's hidden sensations of intense pleasure . . . The G-spot is a woman's prostate gland. When stimulated, it swells with blood and emits ejaculate fluid, usually during orgasm. Author Deborah Sundahl has led seminars on female ejaculation for 15 years, and this book is based on her research. Contents include techniques and positions that help a woman ejaculate, and how men can help their female partners to ejaculate.

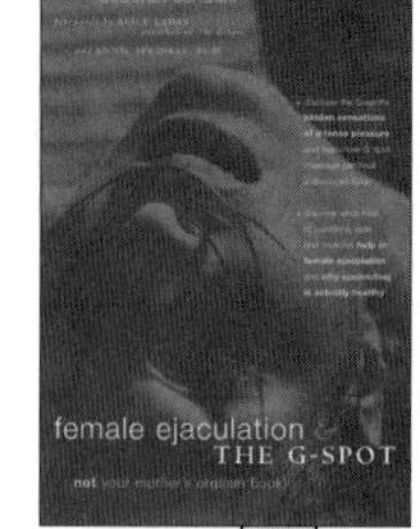

Massage techniques developed by body-work specialists and Tantric healers are also included.

240 pages ... 13 illus. ... Paperback $15.95

TANTRIC SEX FOR WOMEN: A Guide for Lesbian, Bi, Hetero and Solo Lovers

by Christa Schulte

Every woman can enhance her sexual experiences through the use of Tantra. Christa Schulte, a longtime practitioner, introduces women to *Tara-Tantra,* a woman-centered approach that she has developed and taught for many years.

Over 50 exercises are included . . . for solo-lovers, love games for two, rituals, meditations, and massage techniques, all designed to enable women to fulfill their sexual and sensual potential, enrich their relationships, and enjoy the small ecstasies of everyday life. The book will also help men who want to understand women's sexuality and become better partners.

288 pages ... 3 illus. ... 3 b/w photos ... Paperback $15.95

SEXUAL PLEASURE: Reaching New Heights of Sexual Arousal and Intimacy ... Second Edition

To experience deep sexual pleasure, Dr. Keesling explains, you must explore your ability to enjoy basic human touch. Focusing on touch and desire leads to greater passion, sensitivity, and fulfillment for both partners. This book shows how to develop a mastery of one's erotic body. This second edition has material about talking sexy and the unique pleasures of different sexual positions, a new section on oral sex, and 30 new exercises.

264 pages ... 11 illus. ... 14 b/w photos ... Paperback $14.95

Order online at www.hunterhouse.com ... all prices subject to change

More Hunter House Books on SEXUALITY & ORGASM

EXTENDED MASSIVE ORGASM: How You Can Give and Receive Intense Sexual Pleasure *by Steve Bodansky, Ph.D., & Vera Bodansky, Ph.D.*

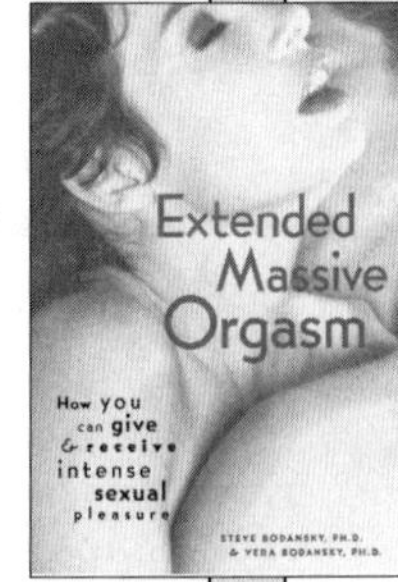

Yes, extended massive orgasms can be achieved! In this hands-on guide to doing it, Steve and Vera Bodansky describe how to take the experience of sex to a new level.

The authors disclose stimulation techniques and uniquely sensitive areas known only to specialized researchers, recommend the best positions for orgasm, and offer strategic advice for every technique from seduction to kissing. With the help of this book you'll find it's never too late — or too early — to make your partner ecstatic in the bedroom.

224 pages ... 5 illus. ... 16 b/w photos ... Paperback $14.95

THE ILLUSTRATED GUIDE TO EXTENDED MASSIVE ORGASM *by Steve Bodansky, Ph.D., & Vera Bodansky, Ph.D.*

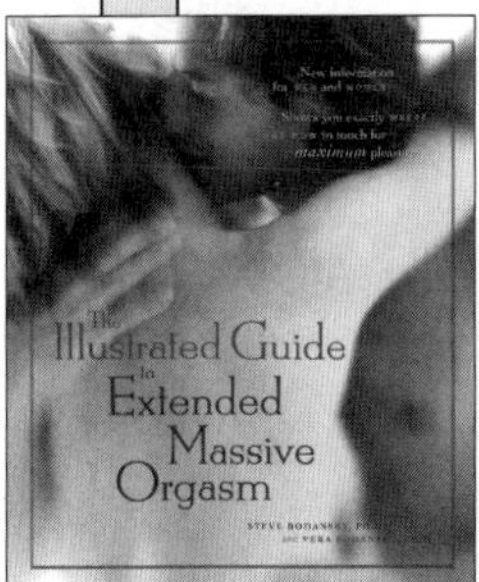

In this companion book, Steve and Vera Bodansky give much more detail about the best hand and body positions for performing and receiving EMO. More than 70 photographs and drawings illustrate genital anatomy and stimulation techniques, and the book covers new ground in the area of male arousal and orgasm.

Suddenly orgasm is no longer just a fleeting moment, but the beginning of lasting arousal that goes far beyond the bedroom.

256 pages ... 57 illus. ... 25 photos ... Paperback $17.95

SIMULTANEOUS ORGASM and Other Joys of Sexual Intimacy *by Michael Riskin, Ph.D., & Anita Banker-Riskin, M.A.*

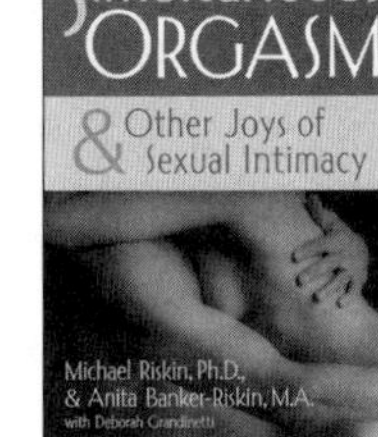

Based on techniques developed at the Human Sexuality Institute, this guide shows couples how they can achieve the special, intimate experience of simultaneous orgasm. The book gives specific techniques and step-by-step instructions that help individuals achieve orgasm separately, and then simultaneously. Exercises include practical advice for relaxing and feeling comfortable with yourself and your partner. A separate section explains the purpose of the exercise and offers insights about how it can positively affect your relationship.

240 pages ... 5 illus. ... 10 b/w photos ... Paperback $14.95

To order or for our FREE catalog or call (800) 266-5592

ORDER FORM

10% DISCOUNT on orders of $50 or more —
20% DISCOUNT on orders of $150 or more —
30% DISCOUNT on orders of $500 or more —
On cost of books for fully prepaid orders

NAME

ADDRESS

CITY/STATE ZIP/POSTCODE

PHONE COUNTRY (outside of U.S.)

TITLE	*QTY*	*PRICE*	*TOTAL*
Sex Secrets of an American Geisha		@ $ 13.95	
Tantric Sex for Women		@ $ 15.95	

Prices subject to change without notice

Please list other titles below:

		@ $	
		@ $	
		@ $	
		@ $	
		@ $	
		@ $	
		@ $	

Check here to receive our book catalog ❑ *FREE*

Shipping Costs

By Priority Mail: first book $4.50, each additional book $1.00
By UPS and to Canada: first book $5.50, each additional book $1.50
For rush orders and other countries call us at (510) 865-5282

TOTAL ______
Less discount @____% (______)
TOTAL COST OF BOOKS ______
Calif. residents add sales tax ______
Shipping & handling ______
TOTAL ENCLOSED ______
Please pay in U.S. funds only

❑ Check ❑ Visa ❑ MasterCard ❑ Discover

Card # ______________________ Exp. date ______

Signature ______________________

Complete and mail to:

Hunter House Inc., Publishers
PO Box 2914, Alameda CA 94501-0914
Website: www.hunterhouse.com
Orders: (800) 266-5592 or email: ordering@hunterhouse.com
Phone (510) 865-5282 Fax (510) 865-4295

SSA 10/2006